PRAISE FOR

The Ocean of Yoga

"Amy Landry's book offers a meaningful compilation of yoga's history and concepts, presented in a way that is both accessible and engaging. I am confident it will serve as a helpful resource and companion for anyone wishing to strengthen their foundation in yoga, whether as a practitioner or a teacher." —PRASAD RANGNEKAR, founder of Yogaprasad Institute

"With context and care to scaffold your practice, *The Ocean of Yoga* generously offers inquiry, depth, respect, and refuge." —ELENA BROWER, bestselling author of *Practice You* and *Hold Nothing*

"Amy Landry's *The Ocean of Yoga* is a luminous guide that takes us beyond the asana into yoga's deeper truth, where philosophy, subtle anatomy, and practice meet in radiant unity. With insight and compassion, Landry honors the sacred lineage while opening up the living wisdom of yoga. Written with clarity, devotion, and depth, this book serves as both a companion for seekers and a resource for teachers. It is a tapestry of knowledge and spirit that reflects the very soul of yoga."—DR. MANASA RAO, yoga educator

"A richly informed guide to yoga and its manifold paths and practices. Landry passionately traces yoga's ancestral roots while carefully delving into the cultural cross-pollination and outcomes of this sacred way of life. *The Ocean of Yoga* is an excellent tome for both practitioners and students to widen their approach to an intuitive form of practice."—MAYA TIWARI, author of *The Path of Practice*

"Amy Landry's *The Ocean of Yoga* is a wonderful handbook for students of yoga. Containing a vast overview of traditions, practices, and terminology, this book will no doubt become a trusted source of yogic knowledge for spiritual seekers to return to again and again."—EDDIE STERN, author, researcher, and founder of Broome Street Yoga

"A passionate reminder that there's much more to yoga than sequences of postures. Amy Landry's approachable primer covers everything from ethics to subtle anatomy, providing signposts for deeper inquiry."—DANIEL SIMPSON, author of *The Truth of Yoga*

"Finally Amy releases the book the yoga community has been waiting for. *The Ocean of Yoga* is a full-spectrum understanding of the science of yoga by a person who doesn't merely study it academically but lives the tradition and keeps it alive by her example."—RAY RAGHUNATH CAPPO, author of *From Punk to Monk* and host of the *Wisdom of the Sages* podcast

"A carefully composed and comprehensive guide to yoga in its most undiluted sense. Equally pedagogical and passionate, this book takes a respectful approach to the historical roots and the many paths of yoga while keeping the reader informed about academic debates on the subject. It is impressive in detail and never sacrifices depth for approachability. Yet it meets the reader where they are, not assuming any previous knowledge, and urges them to reflect on their practice. A skillful synthesis of an enormous subject, this book will take you by the hand and guide you across the great ocean of yoga."—TOVA OLSSON, scholar and author of *Yoga and Tantra*

"Amy has skillfully navigated the vast ocean of yoga with profound depth—much like a submariner—in this charming new book."
—SRIVATSA RAMASWAMI, author of *The Complete Book of Vinyasa Yoga*

"*The Ocean of Yoga* stands out for the clarity with which it presents complex ideas. The book is a carefully woven compilation, seamlessly bringing topics under one umbrella rather than leaving students to gather precious nuggets across different sources. For beginners, it is an invaluable guide to 'connecting the dots,' while for seasoned practitioners, it offers a chance to revisit and deepen their understanding. *The Ocean of Yoga* is what the title promises—vast and timeless."— MINI SHASTRI, founder of Om Yoga Shala

THE OCEAN OF YOGA

A COMPLETE GUIDE TO LIVING THE TEACHINGS, TRADITION & PRACTICE

AMY LANDRY

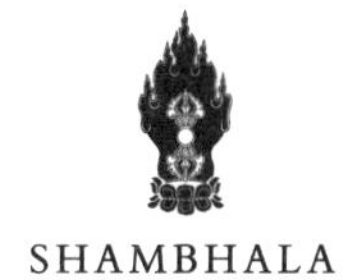

SHAMBHALA

Shambhala Publications, Inc.
2129 13th Street
Boulder, Colorado 80302
www.shambhala.com

Cover art: Tanya Shulga/Shutterstock and mashot/Adobe Stock
Cover design: Daniel Urban-Brown
Interior design: Laura Shaw Design

9 8 7 6 5 4 3 2 1

First Edition
Printed in the United States of America

Shambhala Publications makes every effort to print on acid-free, recycled paper.Shambhala Publications is distributed worldwide by Penguin Random House, Inc., and its subsidiaries.

LIBRARY OF CONGRESS CATALOGING-IN-PUBLICATION DATA
Names: Landry, Amy, author. | Balkaran, Raj, writer of foreword.
Title: The ocean of yoga: a complete guide to living the teachings, tradition, and practice / Amy Landry; foreword by Raj Balkaran.
Description: First edition. | Boulder, Colorado: Shambhala, [2025]
Identifiers: LCCN 2025014716 | ISBN 9781645474692 (trade paperback)
Subjects: LCSH: Yoga. | Yoga—History. | Yoga—Philosophy.
Classification: LCC B132.Y6 L323 2025 | DDC 181/.45—dc23/eng/20250825
LC record available at https://lccn.loc.gov/2025014716

The authorized representative in the EU for product safety and compliance is eucomply OÜ, Pärnu mnt 139b-14, 11317 Tallinn, Estonia, hello@eucompliancepartner.com.

TO MY CHILDREN, WHO HAVE GIVEN ME THE GIFT
OF EXPERIENCING A PROFOUND LOVE LIKE NO OTHER.

TO THE TEACHINGS, AN UNFAILING SOURCE OF SOLACE.

AND TO YOU, THE READER, FOR SEEKING
BEYOND THE SURFACE LEVEL.

सरस्वति नमस्तुभ्यं वरदे कामरूपिणि।
विद्यारम्भं करिष्यामि सिद्धिर्भवतु मे सदा ॥

sarasvati namastubhyam varade kamarupini |
vidyarambham karishyami siddhirbhavatu me sada ||

O Sarasvati, reverential salutations to you, giver of boons
and embodiment of desires in beautiful form,
As these studies commence, may there be success and
accomplishment for me, always.

CONTENTS

FOREWORD

YOGA IS OFTEN PERCEIVED as a physical practice—an exercise, a sequence of postures, and subsequent posturing aimed at ameliorating the body. Yet to dip one's toe into an ocean is to confront its depth, regardless of one's initial perception of it. To those who have journeyed deeper, it becomes evident that yoga is not simply a physical enterprise, but it invariably touches on our emotional, intellectual, and spiritual selves. It is a practice, a philosophy, a way of life, and ultimately a means of spiritual awakening. Yoga spans the gamut of life.

The Ocean of Yoga offers an invitation into this vast aquatic exploration, transitioning from sailing to deep-sea diving. Amy Landry here offers a comprehensive yet accessible guide to the vast intellectual, cultural, spiritual tradition of yoga, one which extends far beyond the mat. Landry skillfully guides us across the waves of history, philosophy, subtle anatomy, and spiritual practice, offering a panoramic yet deeply personal exploration of yoga. She acknowledges the evolving nature of yoga while ensuring that its roots remain honored and intact. Her work reminds us that yoga is neither static nor reducible to any single form—whether physical, philosophical, or devotional—but is instead a confluence of multiple currents leading toward realization.

The book unfolds in five distinct yet interconnected parts. Beginning with an exploration of yoga's historical evolution, Landry guides the reader through the origins and transformations of the practice, illuminating its journey from Vedic times to modern transnational yoga. She then delves into the subtle anatomy of yoga, introducing concepts such as prana, marmas, nadis, and chakras—elements often overlooked in mainstream yoga education. The subsequent sections present the various paths and philosophies of yoga, the essential components of a complete practice, and finally, an exploration of the sacred language and texts that form yoga's foundation.

The modern yoga landscape is one of paradox: never before has yoga been so widely practiced, yet never before have its most essential teachings been so obscured by commercialization and materialism. Many yoga teacher trainings leave students feeling unmoored, disconnected from the deeper roots of the practice, and therefore the deeper layers of their own being. Simultaneously, sincere seekers may find themselves adrift amid the often diluted sea of available information. *The Ocean of Yoga* serves as an antidote to this dilution, offering a structured yet fluid approach to understanding the multidimensionality of yoga. It occupies a crucial and necessary space between yoga's ancient Indian spiritual context and its modern Western evolution. It does not merely recount history or critique modernity; rather, it serves as a bridge, both acknowledging the roots of yoga in its deeply spiritual and philosophical origins while also engaging with the ways it has been reshaped in contemporary practice.

From its origins in the Vedic traditions, the Upanishads, and later the philosophical and Tantrik systems, yoga has always been more than physical movement—it is a comprehensive spiritual discipline aimed at Self-realization, liberation (*moksha*), and the refinement of human consciousness. In the Indian tradition, yoga is inseparable from the larger framework of dharma, the pursuit of inner stillness, and the embodied wisdom of teachers who passed down their knowledge through unbroken lineages. Landry's work deeply respects and upholds these foundations. She brings attention to the *guru-shishya parampara* (teacher-to-student lineage), the role of Vedic and Tantrik influences, and the expansive view of yoga as a multilayered path—including devotion (*bhakti*), knowledge (*jnana*), disciplined action (*karma*), and meditative absorption (*raja yoga*). She also explores the depths of yoga's subtle anatomy, such as vayu, koshas, and the traya sharira, facets that have been historically central but are often omitted in Western yoga spaces.

Yoga's journey into the West has been one of adaptation and, at times, fragmentation. As postural practice (*asana*) became the most visible and marketable aspect of yoga, much of its philosophical and spiritual depth was sidelined. Teacher training programs often prioritize anatomy and sequencing over the transformative teachings of the Yoga Sutras, the Bhagavad Gita, or the Hatha Pradipika. Many practitioners today enter yoga through fitness studios, unaware of its vast philosophical dimensions.

Rather than presenting a binary choice—ancient versus modern, East versus West—*The Ocean of Yoga* encourages an integrated understanding. It invites contemporary students to reconnect with yoga's deeper roots without dismissing its modern expressions. In doing so, it offers a more holistic approach, where practitioners can appreciate yoga's ancient wisdom while also navigating its place in the modern world with discernment.

This book serves as a corrective to the dilution of yoga's richness; indeed, a dip into the ocean beyond the surface, with treasures awaiting therein. It is a companion for those who seek a way to engage with yoga that is both informed by tradition and relevant to contemporary life. It challenges us to practice yoga not just with our bodies but with our whole being—mind, heart, and soul.

What sets *The Ocean of Yoga* apart is its depth and clarity. It is not merely an academic study, nor is it a surface-level manual; rather, it is a living document that invites contemplation, integration, and lifelong inquiry. It provides a foundation for the study of yoga beyond postures, offering a means to cultivate a deeper relationship with the self and others.

For those who yearn to transcend the trappings of Western yoga and delve into its healing and transformative potential, *The Ocean of Yoga* is your diving board. May this book serve as a launchpad for your journey, illuminating the path toward immeasurable wisdom, greater peace, and an abiding experience of the power of the human spirit.

DR. RAJ BALKARAN
Founder of the online Indian Wisdom School
Author of *The Stories Behind the Poses*

THE OCEAN OF YOGA

INTRODUCTION

WITHIN THE VEDIC TRADITION, society has generally turned to both temples and iconography as an access point for devotional worship. To connect with an experience of divinity. This dualistic approach to something godly is often helpful for us, with our human mental faculties.

Metaphorically, *asana* (AH-sa-nuh) are like a main doorway to the temple of yoga. Many enter but overlook the importance of removing their shoes, often leaving with the intention of returning some other time. Some become engrossed in the intricate carvings in the entryway, capturing photos that they may never revisit. Others roam the temple grounds barefoot and eventually get bored or lost. Only a few circumambulate clockwise inside the wondrous temple halls. Rarely do any discover the heart of yoga, resting within the *sanctum*.

You see, with the global explosion of yoga, these days it is easy to find information on whatever commonplace aspect of the practice you desire. Such as any style of postural yoga. Many books readily available offer translations of the most popular yoga philosophy texts. Consider the number of Bhagavad Gita or Yoga Sutra renditions that are available. Without difficulty, you will find innumerable books on breathing, chakras, and meditation. Yet despite the thousands of yoga teacher trainings operating each year around the world, there is still no one stand-alone book that serves as an entry-level guide for students seeking yoga *beyond* the poses and beyond the well-established *Eight Limbs of Yoga*. A budding teacher trainee will receive a manual during their training, yet even the many yoga teacher training manuals are limited and lack the holistic depth of the full spectrum of yoga. Most materials are unable to offer a genuine glimpse into the many facets of the diamond that is yoga.

Additionally, the nature of the modern world has almost entirely removed the traditional lineage-based relationship to a teacher (*guru-shishya parampara*). The nectar of yoga has been far less accessible, or perhaps less relatable, in the context of modern life. Many long for a deep connection to a spiritual teacher, one person who can guide them inward. Our modern society appears hooked on bouncing from one thing or person to another, usually unconsciously, to fill a void. Over many years, it became apparent to me through my in-person and online community that many practitioners experience a lack of certainty or direction. It's concerning how much we appear to have lost our way.

The Ocean of Yoga serves as an accessible and high-level perspective of the mighty path that is yoga. It is a starting point for you as a sincere practitioner to uncover deeper elements of yoga, to go beyond what has been compartmentalized and watered down. This is an invitation to remove your shoes and tread through the doorway to the temple of yoga. In turn, as you roam down ancient hallways, do take time to admire the intricate carvings and embellishments before patiently taking the steps inward to the sanctum. Yoga is a *lifelong* commitment of steady transformation.

Chapter one of this book aims to lay down an important foundation to decode the historical timeline of yoga. We'll uncover the principal periods of the Indian subcontinent that specifically shaped the development of yoga over thousands of years. Much of India's history, as it pertains to yogic practices and philosophies, has been contested at times. Further research and ongoing translations of manuscripts will fill in the gaps and, hopefully, firm up the chronological arrangements. This first part presents critical—yet fascinating—information to provide a student with the basic historical framework and cultural context for their experience of yoga.

In chapter two, we begin to comprehend the subtle yogic anatomy. While for the yoga teacher there is tremendous value in understanding modern or Western anatomy and physiology, there is an immense lack of study and assimilation of the intrinsic approach to the human body within the yogic realm. It is through the knowledge of subtle anatomy that we can further perceive the value of techniques that attempt to penetrate the layers of the self. Chapter two presents the purpose of prana and further explains concepts often glossed over, such as the *kleshas*, *gunas*, *granthis*, and *traya sharira*. Importantly, it clears up confusion around the chakras, which have been considerably modified through the Western lens historically.

With many philosophical systems, styles of postural yoga, cultural customs, and fluid frameworks that guide the various stages of life, it can feel overwhelming to know how best to move forward with yogic pursuits. In chapter three, yoga is presented in the context of being a *path* to be lived rather than a mere set of practices. Chapter four emphasizes key yogic techniques that may form the basis of one's individual *sadhana* (SAH-dha-nuh), applying these progressive practical elements along one's chosen yogic path in a cumulative way. In logical succession, we explore the methods that systematically take us inward. Finally, chapter five brings to light the language of yoga. Here we delve into the beauty of Sanskrit, sacred sound, and the incredibly pertinent texts that literally and metaphorically offer us the timeless wisdom of yoga.

Many students are seeking the nectar of the teachings but don't know where to turn. Many teachers are unsure how to fulfill their responsibility toward yoga. *The Ocean of Yoga* is a guide to lead you into the spiritual heart, into self-inquiry and to a new level of experience that will forever shape you.

This book revealed itself to me as I saw the need for something accessible and affordable that would provide both insight and a sense of relief for serious seekers swimming in the sea of reductionist yoga. There's not one cell in my body that believes I am an expert in any particular area of yoga. However, like a polymath, I hope to have learned, applied, and embodied enough to be able to contribute toward upholding the depths of yoga.

I invite you through thc initial doorway of yoga and encourage you to keep moving inward. You can return to *The Ocean of Yoga* over and over, reading and assimilating differently each time, as you progress and mature on your path of practice. Know that whatever calls you into greater curiosity can carve a path that is uniquely yours. We cannot learn or know everything in one lifetime. No book on yoga could ever be complete, either. You may decide to choose a couple of areas in these pages to dedicate extended time and studentship toward. You may uncover where you are destined to place your wholehearted attention during this lifetime. Guided by the elusive cosmos, may you lead your own adventure into the luminous self within.

There should be no need for a studious practitioner of yoga to spend thousands on teacher training programs to access the knowledge they desire. There should be no need for a dedicated yoga teacher to spend thousands to get qualified on paper only to walk away unfulfilled. Often the content within a teacher training only lightly touches on a few aspects of yoga. In addition, it is difficult to sift through the repetitive onslaught of information being regurgitated online and in books. Again, we can never learn everything about yoga in one lifetime, and it is hard to find the ambrosia. Perhaps this has been for valid reason, such as to minimize the misuse and monetization of the mystical. I've written this book as a guiding tool to spark inquiry and insight and facilitate deeper studies along your path. *The Ocean of Yoga* references multiple systems and aims to create enough clarity for you to move forward with a greater sense of direction and depth.

Yoga is magnificently multifaceted, like a Crown of Light diamond. It is my earnest desire to keep illuminated this diamond that fuels the work you are now reading. My great hope is that *The Ocean of Yoga* will provide a glimmer of the many facets of yoga as both a path and practice.

Let it be known that there is no one tradition, one path, or one approach to yoga. Every day, may we remember that within the walls of a temple we will locate the inner sanctum, and that our body is the same. Yoga is a vehicle to take us inward to the secret chamber where we uncover the warmth and radiant light of the spiritual heart.

Finally, I have learned that we cannot get things right all the time in life. Therefore, the information surrounding any of the teachings, texts, history, and practices shared within these pages could change, especially with the ongoing academic research into yoga. Forgive any errors or misunderstandings. Wholeheartedly, I offer *The Ocean of Yoga*, something I wish had been available to me many years ago and that I hope will land in your hands at the most opportune time. May this be a resource you can reference both now and over years to come, knowing that together we may humbly contribute to upholding the vast richness of yoga.

May your path be dedicated and lifelong. May it always call you into quietude. May you find refuge within the Self.

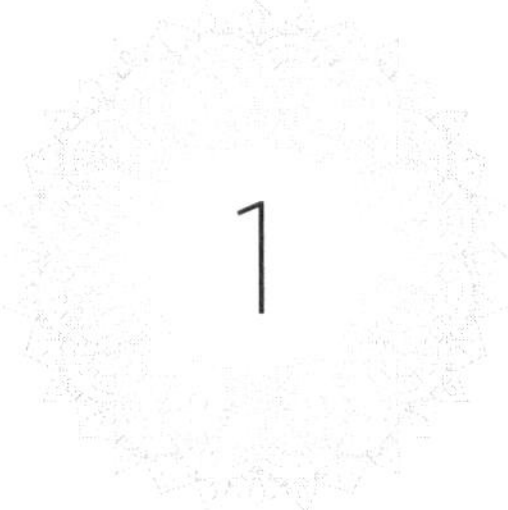

1 THE EVOLUTION OF YOGA

What Is Yoga?

What do we mean when we use the word *yoga* in daily life? We encounter the Sanskrit term in a variety of contexts, including in literature, media, and marketing. Yet, do the connotations we attach to this word resonate with each other, or do they diverge? Many of us never pause to question or actively define our personal understanding of the term, content with the broad definition of "union." Here is a fundamental question: What implications arise for our practice and the future of yoga if we lack this essential clarity? When we say we are "doing" yoga, do we genuinely grasp the essence of our actions, or does it remain elusive? Is it acceptable to accommodate differing meanings? Or is that the point, that yoga does have many meanings that depend on the circumstances and context? These are the inquiries that we shall delve into as we seek a deeper comprehension of the profound practice that is yoga.

A simple and common response to this major question is that yoga is a state of being related to a state of liberation, or union (with the

Supreme or universal consciousness). However, since most of us have never attained a state of realization, how can we possibly understand this elusive quality of being?

The Sanskrit root, *yuj*, often implies yoking, binding, or to join or unify. Perhaps it feels deep and whimsical to think that this meaning reflects a spiritual attainment of sorts. But historically the word *yoga* was used in everyday Indian life outside the context of yoga as we know it. *Yoga* was used to describe the attachment or coupling of an animal, usually a bull, to a cart. It was the harnessing of the animal with a cross-piece. The basic principle here is the act of binding or connecting. It is understood that the word *yoga* in this context was used most often during wartime. Like all Sanskrit words, *yoga* has multiple meanings or translations that depend entirely on the context of its use. The syntax within yogic texts also gives rise to multiple layers of meaning. There is certainly complexity to this inquiry, bearing in mind that language has always evolved with time.

Given that yoga as a spiritual path was originally disseminated through oral tradition, the word was first introduced in written form in the Rigveda. However, it wasn't until the later Upanishads that the word was used more within the context we know today. In Vedic times, yoga was both a means and an aim. In most cases, it had nothing to do with physical positions or practices. Another nuance is to consider the Sanskrit word *yukta*, which is a verb that describes the action of yoga—of yoking.

So, are we best to suggest that yoga is a process, a practice, a path, a form of exercise, a technique, a goal, or a state of being?

Yoga is described by Lord Krishna in the Bhagavad Gita in multiple ways. If you include all variations, such as *yukta* and *yogí*, the word is used over a hundred times within the text, as a noun and verb. One of the more popular interpretations from the Bhagavad Gita occurs when Lord Krishna teaches us that yoga is the art of skillfully performing actions in the world. The context and the commentary of the text are incredibly important when we are trying to grasp the meaning of yoga.

Historically speaking, the meaning of yoga was far from fixed. We can look back to see that in various cases it implied a path of renunciation, contemplation, detachment, abandonment of worldly desires, equanimity, self-remembrance, or the discontinuation of mental afflictions, that is, *nivrtti*. On the other hand, it meant *pravrtti*, applying oneself wholeheartedly to achieve things in the world, being of service to the world and seeking salvation.

With the explosion and commodification of modern yoga globally, the meaning and purpose of the word *yoga* has become alarmingly distorted. Simultaneously, it may be wise to embrace the innovations of yoga. Yoga as a path of practice has continuously evolved over centuries, after all. However, the current developments of the broad yoga tradition are resulting in a slow degradation of its fruitful teachings, despite some beneficial innovations from recent decades. There is no doubt that the current state of the global yoga industry provides great benefit to physical wellness and mental health. But due to capitalist influences and the desire to commodify yoga, sadly the cultural context and subtle teachings of yoga have been drastically diminished. It is we who suffer from this loss. At the very least, yoga should ultimately ignite a withdrawal from external attachment and validation, promoting a state of mind that is steady, discerning, and reflective. In Patanjali's *Yoga Sutra* 1.2, we are told that yoga is the restraint of the fluctuations of the mind: *yogash-chitta-vrtti-nirodha*. This is a timeless teaching, and relevant for practitioners in today's world of chaos and distraction.

The ongoing changes within the global yoga community and industry at large have brought about confusion and conflict. While there is value in adapting some of the teachings to our current worldly climate and ways of life, some traditionalists reasonably believe that to adapt is to dilute, and ultimately add to the deterioration of, the essence of yoga. Perhaps the best way to further contemplate this is to embrace an understanding of the general historical timeline of yoga—at least, as much as we know today, thanks to studious academic research alongside some rare unadulterated transmissions by means of unbroken lineages (*parampara*). Keep in mind that chronological accuracy is challenging and often debated. Nonetheless, one need not be deterred from delving into yoga's past, as it is a key to reviving and retaining the depths of yoga. As more findings are uncovered, some of the following information could be subject to change, especially the order of events. Nevertheless, do embrace ruminations on the history of yoga as a resource for elevating your own studentship.

Lastly, it would be amiss to ignore a question that often plagues the yoga community: Is yoga a religious practice? More specifically, is it a

Hindu practice? The answer is supremely nuanced, but the best starting point to create clarity is to understand the terms *Hindu* and *Hinduism*. Surprising to many, the word *Hindu* is derived from *Sindhu*, which refers to the Indus River. It was originally used as a purely geographical term. When the Persians encountered the Indus Valley civilization, they pronounced *Sindhu* as *Hindu* due to their language's phonetic patterns. Much later, during Islamic colonization and rule in India, the label of *Hindu* came to be used more contrastively, referring to those in India who were not Muslim, and eventually also those who were not Christian, Buddhist, Jain, or Jewish. It was at this time that it became used as a religious and even legal term. During this period of history, Hindus faced heavy taxes, temple destruction, and pressure to convert to Islam, and the label was felt by many to be a marker of second-class citizenship (note the term *dhimmi*).

Eventually, around the time of the British colonial period, the label of "Hinduism" was used to classify and codify Indian traditions, leading to a grouping of many diverse and often contradictory philosophies and practices under what is really an umbrella term. The people themselves preferred, however, the more pertinent term of *Sanatana Dharma*. Sanatana Dharma more appropriately reflects a way of life over any religious ideology. Hinduism does not uphold one God or one scriptural text, like major religions such as Christianity, Islam, or Judaism. In more recent decades, there has been a more empowered renaissance of the label of *Hindu* to revive and defend the wisdom teachings of the Indian subcontinent. It could be said to be used as a unifying identity to counter the control of previous Islamic and British governance. As for yoga, there is no doubt that it is inextricably connected to Sanatana Dharma, for this philosophical way of life was the soil that the seed of yoga sprouted within. Of course, one may argue that this is an oversimplification and does not reflect the complex influences on yoga, which would be reasonable to attest.

How Did We Get Here?

Imagine the history and timeline of the development of yoga as a puzzle with missing pieces. Those missing pieces were most likely destroyed, even lost for eternity, which now creates conflicting ideas around certain developments in the civilization of Bharata—the former name for what is now regarded as the Indian subcontinent, including India and the partitioned Pakistan and Bangladesh, among others. This consideration is a useful foundation for understanding the trajectory of yoga. Many believe that the cultural characteristics and religions of India are exclusively rooted in the Indo-Aryan, and therefore Vedic, traditions. However, there are archaeological discoveries that challenge this. The discoveries indicate that the Indus Valley people had a very established and advanced culture prior, and this included religious and spiritual traits that likely were the original foundation of the Indian culture we know today. Of course, much about the population and life of the Indus civilization is unknown, or yet to be determined. But what we do know is there are no traces of Aryan or Indo-European influence on the Indus people of the time—at least five thousand years ago, possibly up to eight thousand.

The famous Pashupati seal, measuring only 3.56 by 3.53 centimeters and found during the excavation of the ancient city Mohenjo-Daro of the Indus Valley, *potentially* alludes to spiritual practices of the era. It is an estimated 4,000 to 4,500 years old. The main distinguishable form on it is that of a man wearing a horned headdress with multiple adornments, surrounded by mostly herbivorous animals. The human figure on the soapstone seal is in a seated position, which some propose indicates a yogic seat or asana. One such posture is *mulabandhasana*. Mostly due to the symbolism associated with the "lord of animals," Pashupati—a form of the god Shiva (shee-vuh)—it is suggested the figure may be a representation of Shiva himself, hence the name of the seal. It must be said that this is all ultimately speculation and interpretation. For the nature of the ancient Indus Valley lifestyle, to take such a seat would be reasonably natural and commonplace.

You likely get the idea that the origins of the yoga we know today are challenging to ascribe. As previously highlighted, the first written mention of the word *yoga* was in the Rigveda. While various ideas across the four Vedas allude to yoga and influenced the practice, the first descriptions of actual yogic techniques or practices are found in the Upanishads. The Upanishads are the texts, or *shastra* (sh-AH-stra), that evolved from and became the end of the Vedas.

Putting aside the uncertain history and timeline of the ancient people of present-day India, we can see that the nomadic Indo-Aryans likely established across central Asia what we now know as the Vedic tradition. Important to note, the term "Aryan" has tremendously negative connotations globally. This is due to the word having been adopted and adapted by Adolf Hitler and the Nazi Party. Many consider the word to be heavily associated with whiteness and colonization. However, the original use of the word *Aryan* relates to the speakers of Indo-European language who migrated across northern India during the Bronze Age. This was around the same period that the Indus Valley civilization began to decline. Bringing with them their language, which eventually gave rise to Sanskrit, the Aryan people settled over a lengthy period of time. They frequently orchestrated intricate and complex fire ceremonies that were woven into the fabric of daily life. Meanwhile, there is academic unanimity that yoga as a practice of subtle techniques was developing mutually among the ascetics located in northern India. No doubt the ritualistic Vedic ideas and methods influenced these earliest yogis over time, and vice versa.

Renunciation

One could say that the ascetics were the original yogis. Ascetics lived a life of austerity. They were usually depicted naked or near-nude, often with incredibly long hair, like pranic antennae. Renouncing worldly pleasures and attachments, these ascetics may appear to represent nothing like the yoga we know today. However, we know their penances were intended to promote *tapasya*: the cultivation of internal heat, power, or fire. We could say this is much like the internalized ritual of the Hatha and Tantrik paths, which have heavily informed modern yoga. While unproven, it has been speculated that the yoga posture *vrksasana* (vrk-SHAH-suh-nuh) is a modified, householder version of the sadhu's standing on one leg for years or, potentially, an entire lifetime.

As a reflection of their bodily detachments, ascetics often engaged in self-mortification throughout the centuries, such as lying on a bed of nails (as captured by photograph in the 1800s) or sitting in a circle of cow dung fires with the sun raging overhead. There were also practices of fasting, using cannabis, and inverting the body for extended periods. In a simple sense, their discipline was anchored in devotion to a deity (often Lord Shiva) or the Supreme Reality. It was cultivated with the intent to dissolve karma and detach from the individual self as much as possible.

Asceticism is directly and indirectly mentioned in the Vedas alongside indications of the use of various hallucinogenic plants. Additionally, the teachings of Patanjali's Yoga Sutras of the later classical yoga period could have heavily informed the life of an ascetic. While many of the teachings of the Yoga Sutras bring value to and have relevance in our everyday modern lives, ultimately the text does highlight the essential significance of *tapas* (austerity) and promotes both disinterest in the body and detachment from one's mental preferences.

Asceticism also involved the use of variants of cannabis such as bhang and hashish. It would not be uncommon today to walk throughout India and see an ascetic smoking a conical pipe made from clay or stone, called a *chillum*. This act has an association with Shiva, the Lord of Yoga and vanquisher of death. Fast-forward to the development of tantra, and we see that the use of intoxicants was, and still is, one of the defining practices within the "left path" of *vamamarga*, also called *vamachara*. The use of intoxicants is not for the simple purpose of getting high. They are used only for those who have become truly established in self-control and mental stability. For ascetics and tantrikas, the impacts of the intoxicants become an aid to the practice that is being engaged in. In book four of the Yoga Sutras, there is mention of the use of herbs as a means to reveal the veil between the layers of consciousness.

Vedic Culture

Passages that allude to the renunciate lifestyle of ascetics are simply a small part of the vastness of the Vedas themselves. The Sanskrit word *veda* means "knowledge." It is the knowledge of the Vedas that was written down and compiled by the Rishis, the seers. The Vedas are said to contain eternal truths and to have been divinely revealed (*apaurusheya*) to these enlightened sages, rather than composed by them. The four Vedas—Rigveda, Yajurveda, Samaveda, and Artharvaveda—contain extensive philosophical teachings, hymns, mantras, rituals, and incantations. The texts guided society and signified the emergence of Vedic culture and worldview around 2000–3500 years ago at *least*, given this is roughly when they were penned down. The teachings were passed on orally even earlier. This influence included the stature of Brahmin priests, who conducted all the Vedic rituals and held an esteemed place in society, which no doubt had a strong influence on the caste system that still plagues much of India today. Fire ritual as worship, called *homa* or *yajna*, and offerings were notable parts of the daily community life and still endure across India today.

Vedic culture remains a strong aspect of life on the subcontinent, but at its peak it became challenged by a combination of factors. Urban centers bloomed and became more established. Some of the population began to discover and be drawn to other teachings that were spreading across India, such as the Shramana movement, which eventually gave rise to Buddhism and other traditions. The general practices and preferences of ascetics persevered, which resulted in the Brahmins adopting some non-Vedic concepts and ideas. This was likely to maintain their level of influence within communities. Historically, this is when we begin to see cross-pollination of ideas and practices becoming apparent.

It is worth highlighting that the Upanishads, a collection of texts, are considered to be the concluding aspect of the Vedas. As with the Vedas, specific individual authors have not been attributed to the Upanishads, and we learn that they too were divinely revealed to seers who compiled them. The word *upanishad* more commonly translates to "sit down near" (an older additional meaning is "connection"), and the texts were developed as a means of exploring the deeper philosophical and spiritual aspects of existence. They cover topics such as the nature of reality, the individual soul (*atman*), and the ultimate reality (*Brahman*). They formed the philosophical foundation and essence of the Vedanta tradition, one of the six orthodox schools of Indian philosophy. The word *Vedanta* is appropriately translated as "end of the Veda."

Note that the Upanishads each stand on their own, despite being called a collection. The ten to twelve that are considered the most important are referred to as the "major Upanishads." It is within these various shastras that we see a practical sense of yoga mentioned, although not in the way of yoga postures, as we may eagerly anticipate. As an example, within the major *Katha Upanishad* we uncover the practice of withdrawing the senses, which is mentioned multiple times both literally and metaphorically. Across the various Upanishads, we read of concentration; the layered sheaths (often called *koshas*) of the body; subtle anatomy containing numerous *nadis*; breath as prana; and the various *vayus*, or directions of pranic movement. It is surprising the Upanishads are not more heavily emphasized or embraced for study by yoga practitioners or teachers, given that they provide seemingly small but significant insights into the earliest developments of yoga, historically speaking. With that in mind, we will shed a little more light on them later in the book.

Classical Yoga

Fast-forward along the timeline and we come to another meaningful and noteworthy text: the Mahabharata, written around 400 B.C.E. to 400 C.E. Considered an *itihasa* (a historical narrative, *as it happened*, and one that also conveys deeper truths), the Mahabharata is traditionally attributed to the sage Vyasa, who is said to be responsible for this collection of stories that uphold a larger overarching narrative. The more commonly known and studied Bhagavad Gita is a part of this Indian epic and technically not a stand-alone text in isolation. Considered one of the foundational texts of yoga philosophy, the Bhagavad Gita conveys an abundance of definitions of yoga throughout its dialogues and storyline. However, yoga is woven throughout several other sections of the Mahabharata also. The epic certainly had a lasting impact on society and continues to influence Indian culture. It presents the reader with moral dilemmas, ethical choices, customs, and conduct. It also presents ideas of political governance and philosophical discourse, promotes artistic and cultural expression, and alludes to the significance of women (amid a real-life patriarchal society at the time). Ultimately, the Mahabharata played a pivotal role in shaping the moral, social, and philosophical fabric of ancient Indian society with the development of yoga as a path of practice. It has directly informed the paths of Bhakti and Karma yoga, offering any householder a framework for living daily life, presenting the practical concepts of the four *purushartha*.

Following, the period of classical yoga started to swell. The teachings of classical yoga, also called Raja yoga, continue to be foundational to and influential in most modern mainstream yoga practices. They were unquestionably popularized in the Western world in much later times by Swami Vivekananda. But without jumping ahead, we must acknowledge a widely acclaimed text: Patanjali's Yoga Sutras. This manual comprises four chapters, or *pada* (PAH-duh), each broken into many small sutras, or lines. The Yoga Sutras text is not only the basis of the classical yoga philosophy, but additionally, the text is heavily, though not entirely, informed by Samkhya philosophy. Alongside the previously mentioned Vedanta, Samkhya (a dualistic path) is one of the six orthodox *darshana*, or schools of Indian philosophy. In fact, it is one of the oldest codified philosophical systems of India, and some of its elements are woven throughout the Mahabharata.

Although the dates are disputed, it is generally believed Patanjali's Yoga Sutras was penned between the second century B.C.E. and the fifth century C.E. This shastra, or sacred scripture, outlines an eightfold path of yoga (Ashtanga yoga) as a systematic guide for practitioners to attain Self-realization. It is not to be confused with the physically demanding modern style of ashtanga vinyasa yoga popularized by Sri K. Pattabhi Jois (1915–2009).

Patanjali's eight-limbed path consists of ethical and moral principles (*yama* and *niyama*), physical postures (*asana*), breath control (*pranayama*), sensory withdrawal (*pratyahara*), concentration (*dharana*), meditation (*dhyana*), and the state of profound meditative absorption (*samadhi*). These eight auxiliaries are heavily studied and promoted in today's modern yoga landscape. However, they form only a small component of the Yoga Sutras text at large. Chapters 1 and 2 of the entire text seem to be the most common and easy to dissect. There are many commentaries on the Yoga Sutras, most being presented for a modern audience. Despite being a pivotal text for the modern yoga practitioner, Patanjali's Sutras place only a minuscule focus on yoga posture. The teachings on asana that have been presented are ultimately for their original purpose, which is to prepare the body to sit (and thus settle)—that is, to meditate. Perhaps the text holds more parallels to the inward-focused path of a meditator or an ascetic than to a hot power vinyasa practitioner. The Yoga Sutras also presents us with the contemplation of separation and *not* union. Patanjali encourages us to approach liberation (*kaivalya*) through the realization that the true individual Self is separate from all that is perceived. He is guiding us to the disentanglement of *purusha* (unchanging, eternal, pure consciousness) from the influence of *prakriti* (the material, manifest world and all its activities experienced through the mind and senses).

Patanjali also illuminates for us teachings on mental afflictions, or kleshas. These five torments of the mind are what obstruct our progress on the path of yoga, along with the unfolding of our individual karma. Patanjali encourages self-discipline and practice, self-inquiry through reading scripture, and unwavering devotion to Ishvara (the omnipresent Supreme) as the means to uproot and remove mental impressions. Especially the deep-rooted *vasana* (VAH-suh-NAH) that are the basis of our conditioning and tendencies. Not all vasanas (sometimes likened to *samskara*) are bad. Some have the potential to steer us toward virtuous actions. This leads us to the foundational approach of the eight-limbed path, the *yama* and *niyama*. The yamas are five ethical observances. The niyamas are five self-disciplines. These offer guidelines for everyday life. For living yoga, you could say. They have become somewhat of a backbone for how yoga practitioners aspire to conduct themselves in all circumstances and relationships in society.

The yamas and niyamas were no doubt intended to be more austere than we see them in today's world. The ten recommendations are indisputably open to interpretation nowadays. For example, today *ahimsa* often refers to the choice of a plant-based diet. However, in Vedic times Brahmin priests commonly used cows for sacrifice; that is, until the later influence of both Buddhism and Jainism. The more unorthodox path of Tantra has often involved the consumption of meat and continues to do so. Nonetheless, the yamas and niyamas provide immense value and structure for those who desire to expand their application of yoga into each moment.

Interestingly, Patanjali's Yoga Sutras generally call upon *vairagya* (detachment or dispassion) and a withdrawal from the world. Meanwhile, the Bhagavad Gita encourages the opposite: for us to be skillfully in the world and actively engaging with it. This is why the complexities and nuances continue. Putting aside the consideration that the text is seemingly directed more toward a life of renunciation, it is worthwhile noting that the Yoga Sutras has not always been the most approved, let alone a celebrated, compilation of teachings. Patanjali had his critics. Adi Shankara, an eighth-century South Indian philosopher, theologian, and scholar, was one of them. Adi Shankaracharya is known as one of the most important figures in the history of the Advaita Vedanta (nondualistic) tradition. It is suggested that, around 1200 C.E., Patanjali's Yoga Sutras may have fallen out of common use, although this is disputed. That aside, given that the Yoga Sutras was one of the first yoga-related

Indian texts to be translated from Sanskrit to English, in the early 1900s, it understandably garnered enormous global interest. It made the ancient teachings of yoga accessible to the wider English-speaking world, and it therefore played a significant role in spreading the knowledge of yoga to the West.

The Body as a Temple

Yoga becomes more practical, physical, and postural when expressed later through the Tantrik and Hatha movements. Today Tantra is commonly misunderstood both within India and beyond. It is thought to be a form of black magic or sorcery (in the East), or about sex (in the West). The reality is that Tantra has informed modern yoga far more than most know. The word *tantra* has many meanings. A common one is "to loom." The root *tan* generally translates to "weave," "expand," and "extend." *Tra* translates to "tool" or "instrument" (as in the word *mantra*). We could suggest that Tantra is a secular path. It is valuable to understand that it offers multiple pathways or systems. It is not a single unified tradition. A simplistic example would be to highlight the existence of Hindu, Jain, and Buddhist Tantra. All Tantrik paths have always seen the human body as a temple, to be honored and worshipped. Tantra recognizes one's individuality and personality. The Tantrik approach is to go through the body to transcend the body. This is unlike other yogic paths, which continue to promote disidentification with the individual human form.

Sometime from the fifth century C.E. onward, Tantra began to spread and gained rapid importance. Many suggest that it had been practiced and passed down by oral tradition, like the Vedic teachings, for many years prior. While there is no evidence yet, some claim Tantra dates back to the Indus Valley civilization. Regardless, Tantra very likely pulled some influence from the Vedas. What underpinned all Tantrik systems was the use of both external and internal ritual. Developing gradually over centuries, Tantra advocated for maintaining a relationship with worldly life and the elements. It provided tools easily accessible to the householder. While many Tantrik practices were elaborate, elusive, and esoteric, we can easily see the use of mantra, meditation, mystical symbolic *yantra*, and the subtle yogic anatomy as central components that are still woven through modern yoga.

In Tantra, the yogic body contains the entire universe in microcosmic form. It is where we learn of the nadis, the granthis, and the chakras. At its peak, Tantra had dual and nondual paths that emphasized the worship of Shiva and Shakti (shuk-tee)—the masculine and feminine forces. Aside from the widely misunderstood unorthodox systems, for the average person Tantra invited into the home a sense of devotional celebration toward daily life. It also inspired more detailed depictions of the deities in statues and imagery alongside the development of temples.

Rising around the ninth to tenth centuries C.E., Hatha yoga emerged as a distinctly more postural and physical path than ever seen prior. Hatha yoga certainly borrowed and adapted elements of Tantra but was also heavily influenced by the penances and practices of the ascetics. It is ultimately a hybrid. Tantra and Hatha yoga are equally misunderstood. Ask the average yoga practitioner or teacher, and they will likely state that "hatha" is a gentle and more static style of postural yoga. However, Hatha yoga is a path or tradition. Alongside yoga postures, it encompasses other elements of yoga such as pranayama and meditation. The tradition also includes the six cleansing techniques, called *shatkriya*. To be immersed in Hatha yoga (sometimes Hathayoga) is to choose a dynamic path—the Sanskrit word *hatha* translates to "force"—that includes applying consistent restraint. Many of the practical aspects of Hatha yoga were modified from the intense ascetic austerities and presented to be applicable and useful for the average householder.

Most Hatha-related texts do not mention doctrine as much as practice and techniques. The most widely known text is the Hatha Pradipika (also Hathayogapradipika) attributed to Svatmarama. Many related texts that were translated much later (some very recently) appear to offer further insight into Hatha yoga, such as the *Amaraugha*, *Dattatreya Yoga Shastra*, *Yoga Taravali* (TAH-RAH-va-lee), and the *Hathatattvakaumudi*, as a small sample. Many of the texts provide specific conditions under which it is and is not advised to practice. This includes location, time of day, and state of the body. They emphasize pranayama, mudra, bandha, and the anatomy of the subtle body such as the nadis and kundalini. If Hatha were a *style* of postural yoga, it would be essential to teach and practice all these elements within an everyday yoga class.

The initial propagators of Hatha yoga are believed to be Matsyendranatha and his highly revered disciple, Gorakhanatha. The techniques of

Hatha yoga were fundamentally intended to prepare the body for meditation and higher spiritual states. Therefore, as Hatha gained popularity over the centuries, it was practiced by yogis and ascetics who sought to achieve bodily resilience as an aid to their spiritual pursuits. The Nath yogis in particular were at their height between the fourteenth and seventeenth centuries C.E. Unbroken Hatha lineages are still alive in present-day India and Nepal. They are widely regarded as a part of the cultural and spiritual landscape.

Cross-Pollination

The seventeenth century marked the arrival of the British into India. It was around this period that we can affirm at least eighty-four yoga postures were described and taught across various Hatha yoga manuals. A figure of over one hundred is likely much more accurate. Many of the Sanskrit names of the postures differ to those same postures we know and practice in modern yoga. Across the span of British governance, Hatha yoga experienced a notable decline after the ascetics appeared to give up their revolt against the British Raj. This decline was alongside many of the timeless traditions of India, including the arts. The British regarded the yogis as perhaps sinister and most certainly preposterous and obscene.

Colonial rule peaked in the late eighteenth to the nineteenth century. During this period, in 1875, the Theosophical Society was formed in the United States. Despite the oppression of yogic teachings and lifestyle across India, the Theosophical Society founders traveled to and set up a base in Chennai. In turn, they played a significant and pivotal role in introducing and popularizing Indian philosophies among a Western audience. It is important to note that the teachings they shared were filtered through their cultural lens. As a result, they directly modified some concepts within yoga, such as the chakra system, into how we in the West know them at present.

Swami Vivekananda's subsequent visits to the United States strongly contributed to the globalization of yoga and Indian philosophies. The earliest was in 1893, when he delivered the eloquent "Chicago Speech" at the first-ever Parliament of the World's Religions. Advocating for tolerance, his famous speech is regarded by many as truly iconic. He emphasized the universality of spiritual truths, urging us to embrace diversity while recognizing the unity beneath all. In Vivekananda's revered discourses, he pressed that yoga transcended the boundaries of physical practice. Swami Vivekananda himself was a chief disciple of the nineteenth-century saint Sri Ramakrishna.

Established in England in the mid-nineteenth century, the YMCA physical culture movement expanded globally, and in the mid-1800s it found its place within India, setting up in Kolkata. It played a significant role in shaping Indian health practices and sports in the decades following, quickly contributing to the development of organized physical education in the country. European countries continued to spread their influence on fitness, resulting in exercise classes finding their way into Indian communities and school classrooms at the same time that competitive sports were rising in popularity throughout the subcontinent.

Pioneers of Modern Yoga

Meanwhile, starting around the 1920s, early pioneers of modern yoga such as Sri Tirumalai Krishnamacharya began developing and expanding the number of yoga postures, specifically standing postures. Krishnamacharya, often known as the "father of modern yoga" was a Sanskrit scholar and qualified Ayurvedic physician as well as a devotional man. He spent many years studying Sanskrit and the six darshanas, or schools, of Indian philosophy.

Krishnamacharya claimed to have found a guru, Yogeshwara Ramamohana Brahmachari, who lived deep in the Himalaya, in a cave beyond Nepal. Krishnamacharya told his students that his studies with Ramamohana Brahmachari continued throughout seven and a half years and included both physical and philosophical aspects of yoga. Much of Krishnamacharya's story of this time is not confirmed, and academic research has uncovered contradictions. Regardless, his knowledge and expertise were sufficiently evident at the time that the maharaja of Mysore sought him out in Varanasi in the 1920s. Krishnamacharya went to teach the maharaja and his family at the Mysore palace. It was during this time that he gave many public demonstrations of the yoga he was continuing to develop and evolve.

Krishnamacharya solidified his influence within the local community, and after an invitation to teach at the Sanskrit College of Mysore in 1931, the maharaja asked him to establish a yoga school at the nearby Jaganmohan Palace, which opened in 1933. Shortly afterward, he wrote and published the book *Yoga Makaranda*. It is argued that Krishnamacharya was influenced by the Mysore palace gymnasts and other yoga pioneers of the time who wove an influence of the physical culture movement into their presentation of yoga. Impressively, Krishnamacharya went on to live to a hundred years of age, which was no doubt influenced by his unwavering dedication to the yoga practice and his knowledge of Ayurveda. Krishnamacharya was undoubtedly a significant figure in the modern yoga movement overall, as we will uncover further on. In large part, this is thanks to a handful of his key students who brought yoga to the global arena in the decades following.

Born in 1883, Swami Kuvalayananda spearheaded research into understanding yoga from a scientific point of view from 1920 onward. Spiritually minded and driven, Kuvalayananda had an extensive influence on the evolution of yoga as exercise. He set up multiple branches of his Kaivalyadhama Health and Yoga Research Centre across India to study the physiology of various practical aspects of yoga, such as asana, pranayama, bandha, mudra, and kriya. Around the same period, Kuvalayananda established *Yoga Mimamsa* (mee-MAHM-sah), a journal publishing scientific research and experiments within the field. Impressively, *Yoga Mimamsa* is an active quarterly publication even to this day.

Swami Sivananda Saraswati was a proponent of yoga throughout India. Born under the name of Kuppuswami in 1887 into a devotional and religious household, he went on to complete medical school and pursue a career as a medical doctor. After working abroad for a decade in what is now Malaysia, in 1924 he returned to his homeland of India to pursue a spiritual yearning. It was in Rishikesh that Sivananda met his guru, Vishvananda Saraswati in 1925. He was initiated into the Sannyasa order shortly afterward. Over the years he maintained a steadfast commitment to supporting the ill while devoting lengths of time to rigorous penances. He established the Divine Life Society in 1936 and went on to author numerous books. Sivananda relentlessly promoted Vedanta and other philosophical teachings to the general public across India for decades, but he was not without his critics.

Sivananda had several disciples who went on to continue his legacy, including the global expansion of his teachings. The most prominent is Satyananda Saraswati, who founded the Bihar School of Yoga (and who, despite his passing in 2009, has recently come under fire with significant controversy). Through the Bihar School of Yoga, the traditional system of Satyananda yoga has spread globally through the expansion of many ashrams and yoga teacher training programs. Another central disciple of Sivananda was Swami Satchidananda Saraswati, who founded the Integral Yoga Institute. Satchidananda opened one of the institute's branches in the United States in 1970 after he traveled abroad to share the teachings and speak at the 1969 Woodstock Festival. He became a U.S. citizen in 1976.

Finally, Vishnudevananda Saraswati was another important disciple of Sivananda. Vishnudevananda was perhaps most known for disseminating the more practical and physical aspects of yoga, those of asana and pranayama, from his teacher. In his early twenties he was initiated into the Sannyasa order, and less than a decade later he was traveling across the United States teaching Hatha yoga with an emphasis on asana, pranayama, shatkriya, and a sattvic vegetarian diet. Due to this, we now have the style called Sivananda yoga. It was Vishnudevananda who introduced yoga to George Harrison of the Beatles in the 1960s when the band was in Rishikesh to further study Transcendental Meditation with Maharishi Mahesh Yogi.

Born Mukunda Lal Ghosh in 1893, Paramahamsa Yogananda is most renowned around the world due to his pivotal book, *Autobiography of a Yogi*. Spiritually inclined, in his late teenage years Yogananda became a chief disciple of Sri Yukteswar Giri, who was a direct disciple of the remarkable Lahiri Mahasaya. After graduating from college, Yogananda took direct vows of initiation into the monastic order. This lineage became the most well-known of Kriya yoga worldwide. At age twenty-seven Yogananda was sent by Sri Yukteswar to emigrate to America, making him the first Indian teacher to settle in the United States. Here he founded the Self-Realization Fellowship to disseminate the teachings of his Kriya yoga tradition. This was an extension of his Yogoda Satsanga Society, which he established in India in 1917. *Autobiography of a Yogi* was first published in 1946 (the year before India's independence), and it went on to have massive worldwide influence. It is still one of the foremost books on yoga, influencing practitioners globally. Some may even suggest that reading and assimilating the book is a crucial initiation, of a kind, for the modern yoga practitioner who is seeking greater insight on their path.

Bishnu Charan Ghosh, born in 1903, grew up with the influence of Kriya yoga within his home life. Ghosh was the younger brother of the prominent Paramahamsa Yogananda. Their parents were students of Lahiri Mahasaya, after all. It was Yogananda who first taught Ghosh various shatkriya techniques and yoga asanas that were associated with Hatha yoga at the time. Ghosh held an unwavering dedication to physical health and well-being, and at age twenty he founded the College of Physical Education in Kolkata, which is now run by his granddaughter. Ghosh was both a bodybuilder and a Hatha yogi. He developed Ghosh yoga, a system of practices influenced by Yogananda's Yogoda system of techniques as well as his own interest in and experience with physical culture.

The Ghosh yoga approach is regarded as therapeutic for both the body and mind. While very physical, it is anchored in the values of traditional yoga. The Ghosh yoga process is characterized by its use of stillness in *shavasana* (the supine "corpse posture") between postures. Its approach is similar to that of physical therapy and was taught on an individual and prescriptive basis. Two of Ghosh's students continued the legacy, adding to the popularization of yoga worldwide. One was Buddha Bose. The other was the infamous Bikram Choudhury, who later introduced the physically intense, one-size-fits-all Bikram yoga sequence when he brought yoga to the West in the 1970s.

The Transnational Landscape

Krishnamacharya produced several students who went on to shape the landscape of yoga. K. Pattabhi Jois, born in 1915, started studying with his teacher at a young age in the late 1920s and continued for several years. After a short time, he began to develop his own distinct style and was teaching in Mysore from the 1930s onward. Pattabhi Jois refined his ashtanga vinyasa yoga system, often called Mysore-style yoga, and opened the Ashtanga Yoga Research Institute at his own home in Mysore in 1948. His dynamic and adjustment-heavy approach to yoga asana became wildly popular with students traveling from around the globe to study intensively at the Institute each year. Pattabhi Jois published his first book, *Yoga Mala*, in 1962. Two years later, a hall had to be built to accommodate the growing number of students. Jois held and maintained the traditional apprenticeship approach as a means to formally authorize his students to teach the signature Mysore-style method.

Preserving the ashtanga vinyasa tradition, Sharath Jois, the grandson of Pattabhi Jois, has overseen the institute since his passing in 2009. However, Sharath also passed away in November 2024 unexpectedly, at age fifty-three, which rocked the community. Historically, the Mysore-style approach is the first we see where postures are linked in a type of flowing sequence. Undoubtedly, this style of yoga asana has heavily influenced the vigorous modern mainstream styles, such as Power Vinyasa yoga, that are everywhere today. This may well be due to Jois's extended international visit to California in the 1970s.

Another substantially influential student of Krishnamacharya was B.K.S. Iyengar. Iyengar, who was born in 1918 and spent years severely ill as a child, was pivotal in shaping the alignment-focused and prop-heavy approach to yoga asana. Interestingly, Iyengar studied directly with Krishnamacharya for only approximately three years, beginning in 1934. Iyengar's innovative approach consisted of using the expanding catalogue of asanas he learned from Krishnamacharya and maintaining a therapeutic interest by weaving in props as physical aids. The *initial* purpose of props appears to have been so that students could grasp a greater awareness of their bodies within a posture before progressing to performing it without support. Interestingly, while we have Iyengar to thank for his diversity, creativity, and depth in utilizing a huge variety of props, physical aids have been used in yoga for centuries at least. An example would be the strap. Seen in sculptures and paintings, this belt (sometimes made from a cloth strip and called a *yogapatta*) was used wrapped around the lower back and legs while in a seated position. Another example is using a stick or *stambha*, usually T-shaped, where the hands are placed on it to assist the body and spine to remain erect when seated during meditation. With a reputation as a disciplinarian, Iyengar likened the asana to an active meditative state. The static and intense nature of the style no doubt brought on sharp concentration.

Iyengar began traveling internationally to promote yoga in the 1950s, teaching, by request of his hosts, an approach that touted benefits related only to physical health and wellness. In 1966 the English-language version of Iyengar's renowned book *Light on Yoga* was published. He went on to open the Ramamani Iyengar Memorial Yoga Institute in Pune, India, in 1975. Iyengar was also known to teach and strongly advocate for pranayama techniques, and he published *Light on Pranayama* in 1981. Like Pattabhi Jois, Iyengar always maintained the traditional apprentice-style model for approving his students to teach. Sustaining an inspiring dedication to his personal practice, Iyengar passed away in 2014 at the age of ninety-five.

Born Eugenie Peterson in the Russian Empire in 1899, Indra Devi was nicknamed the "First Lady of Yoga." Fascinated with India, she spent several years traveling to the subcontinent from age fifteen, while building her profile as a performer. Through a fortunate connection to the maharaja of Mysore, Devi became the first female student of the esteemed Krishnamacharya. She spent more than a handful of years in the 1930s with Krishnamacharya before taking yoga to China very briefly, then opening a yoga school in Hollywood in the 1940s. Devi presented yoga to Hollywood celebrities to alleviate stress and anxiety, popularizing it as a holistic practice for body and mind. She packaged it in a way that wove yoga with Western sensibilities. Indra Devi, one of the first females to bring yoga to the West, passed away in 2002 at age 102.

A Change in Governance

In 1947, one hundred years after the YMCA arrived, the British Raj ended and India gained independence once again. Hatha yoga began to regain a greater prominence. As India developed its identity over the years following independence, so too did yoga. This evolution of yoga was more rapid than ever before. India embraced the global trend of valuing physical exercise training for the sake of bodily health and started to recoup its rich spiritual identity.

T.K.V. Desikachar was one of Krishnamacharya's sons and most prominent students. Born in 1938, Desikachar learned yoga from childhood and throughout his entire life, thanks to his father. Desikachar was exposed to Krishnamacharya's wealth of knowledge across many areas, including Sanskrit, Vedic chanting, and Ayurveda. He learned both the physical and philosophical aspects of yoga. Desikachar's approach to teaching yoga later in life was heavily influenced by his father's therapeutic method of adapting yoga to the individual. Desikachar is often credited as being one of the first proponents (if not the first) of formalized yoga therapy (*yoga-cíkitsa*). His approach, widely known as Vini yoga, was to prescribe yoga practices according to the needs and conditions of each unique person. In 1976 Desikachar established the Krishnamacharya Yoga Mandiram (KYM) Yoga Center in Chennai to preserve the invaluable teachings of his father. Desikachar published his influential book *The Heart of Yoga: Developing a Personal Practice* in 1995. It is commonly used worldwide as a resource for yoga teacher training. The renowned KYM center has continued to offer a wealth of programs, workshops, and activities over the decades following its inception. Desikachar passed away in 2016 at age seventy-eight.

Another respected teacher in our modern yoga climate, Srivatsa Ramaswami studied under the guidance of Krishnamacharya for over three decades. Born in 1939, Srivatsa Ramaswami began his studies under his teacher in the late 1950s. Known for his dedication to preserving and transmitting the teachings he received from Krishnamacharya, Ramaswami teaches a style developed directly from his studies called *vinyasa krama*. The approach encompasses a slow, methodical breath-based linking of asanas and an emphasis on the importance of pranayama, philosophy, mantra, and meditation. The asanas include *surya namaskar* (sun salutation) and are categorized into various set sequences that can be practiced in isolation or together, depending on the ability of the practitioner. Having authored four books, Ramaswami has continued to travel extensively between India and the United States over many years to teach. Considerably, he was one of the longest-standing students of the acclaimed Krishnamacharya, making Ramaswami a crucial link to one of the most significant authorities of modern yoga developments.

A. G. Mohan, born in 1945, was another later and long-term student of Krishnamacharya. He and his wife, Indra Mohan, commenced their studies under their teacher in 1971, continuing until Krishnamacharya's passing. Mohan became the honorary secretary of the aforementioned Krishnamacharya Yoga Mandiram from 1976 until 1989. Aside from yoga, Mohan pursued studies in fields such as Ayurveda and *Jyotisha* (Vedic astrology) and authored seven books, including a translation of the important Yoga Yajnavalkya text. He and his wife are two of the few who received postgraduate diplomas in yoga from Krishnamacharya himself. Together they went on to co-create Svastha Yoga and Ayurveda, the respected banner under which they offer authentic and traditional knowledge through various programs, holding an ongoing emphasis on yoga therapy. Their two children, Dr. Ganesh Mohan and Nitya Mohan, also offer their skills and experience by facilitating trainings through Svastha Yoga and Ayurveda.

Amalgamation

Yoga has transformed quickly and dramatically throughout the twentieth century. The physical developments of postural yoga were shaped by a synthesis of Hatha yoga techniques, European gymnastics and physical culture, bodybuilding, wrestling, and military calisthenics. Likely, there was also an influence by traditional South Indian martial arts along with the revival of dance forms that were codified and later recognized as Classical by the Indian government. Until recently, it appears that the postural yoga practice was always paired with other therapeutic elements and philosophical teachings. Knowledge of Sanskrit and Ayurveda was commonplace in society and woven through the practice on some level.

While yoga has always been evolving and has never been represented by just one tradition or lineage, the current state of yoga globally is ghastly diluted. The association with yoga as fitness has amplified. The word *yoga* has come to signify physical exercise exclusively. Meditation is seen as something separate from yoga. The popular breathwork trend has been mostly disconnected from its pranayama roots. "Advanced" yoga is seen to be associated primarily with complex, challenging, and out-of-reach-for-most postures, many of which are performed by those who come from a background in gymnastics or the like.

Yoga has become wildly commodified, commercialized, and compartmentalized, even within parts of India. Yoga teachers are perceived as successful based on their community size and social media fame. Anyone with the money can embark on a yoga teacher training program without any personal practice under their belt. Public yoga classes are commonly presented in unison with an entirely unrelated activity, as in "beer yoga" or "goat yoga." How these could take anyone inward, closer to the state of yoga, is impossible to see. Historically, yoga has been a melting pot of ideas and methodologies that have only more recently been sectionalized and cherry-picked, leaving a watered-down facade of the timeless path. Ironically, as a result, we now see "yoga" being intermingled with other trends, which does nothing to close the gaps among the essential ingredients that fundamentally unite to offer us the nectar of yoga.

As one reflects on the historical junctures, it becomes evident that yoga has continued to adapt to and evolve with society. It is important that this is understood and that we do not start to police the current outlook. Meanwhile, we absolutely must ensure that the essence of yoga is not trampled upon. We must safeguard the sanctity of yoga. In a world where asana has become addictive and so many are uncomfortable with stillness and silence, it appears we are often only reinforcing this habitual disposition. To earnestly experience the benefits of yoga, there must be a maturity with and beyond the postures, particularly the way we perform and integrate them.

Modern transnational yoga is of value in our world right now. It is true that the posture-dominant approach is incredibly helpful to the modern body. The modern body has become riddled with discomfort and disease due to our luxuries and sedentary lifestyles. The postural practice assists in promoting better movement and mobility, improves sleep and strength, and aids us in beginning to unravel emotional trauma and conditioning. Many of us have experienced the emotional outpour while in a seated hip-opening pose or a supine prop-supported backbend.

We know this postural yoga makes us feel good, yet the majority rarely go beyond this physical practice. Is it due to our superficial attachments to the body? Are we afraid to slow down enough to face the depths of our mind, or even our impatience? Are we terrified of the unknown and our patterned responses or our true nature? Asana is a path with richly transformative practices. The Sanskrit word *asana* means "to sit," after all. Surely an advanced practice is one where we become more comfortable with stillness. One where we choose quality of asana over quantity through an invitation into stillness within the postures—and not only the restorative ones. An advanced postural practice, in the truest sense, integrates more inwardly oriented aspects of asana itself, such as bandha and mudra, that work with the subtle yogic anatomy. And what about the practices that require absolutely no formal postures at all—pranayama and mantra, for example?

It is borderline impossible to find something we could call unadulterated yoga. Within the Indian subcontinent, over thousands of years, many practices and methods have been shared among the Buddhists, Shaivites, and Jains, for example. In today's world, many are unaware that Hindu is an umbrella term and not one individual religion. There has always been some kind of intermingling within both spiritual and religious systems. But the question is, have we now gone too far?

Where to from Here?

Curiosity and critical thinking are pivotal. How can we preserve yoga and embrace its evolution? Who decides how it unfolds from here? Billions of dollars are spent annually on yoga accessories and attire, fueling further attachment and driving greater distance from the heart of the practice. Yoga gurus in India and the West continue to fall from grace after revelations of ongoing abuse and exploitation of students. The arguments continue over what is (mis)appropriation versus appreciation of yoga. Who owns yoga, and is it religious? Can credibility and authenticity regarding yoga be automatically attributed to South Asian ethnicity? What is authentic yoga anyway? Is yoga political? Does yoga have an agenda? What if we don't all agree? What constitutes a readiness to teach others? Is it appropriate to translate ancient teachings in our own personal way without much regard for the original meaning nor the context it was written in? Do we find a teacher and then surrender to their tradition, or is this disempowering? Navigating these sorts of questions may feel hopeless at times. There are certainly tensions around all these issues. Yet, yoga aims to teach us dispassion and detachment. So, do we let it all go, free ourselves of any concern, withdraw from the world, and simply do the practice? Or do we engage outwardly to pursue dharma, enjoy worldly benefits, and as a result positively impact the progress of yoga within our community? Can we do both?

It may not appear to be the case when we look around, but yoga is more about the way we live our lives than what we do in structured time on a rubber mat. As this book aims to uncover, there are multiple facets of yoga to engage in. Therefore, one could be a sincere *sadhaka* (SAH-dhu-kuh) with zero postural practice. Some modern-day yoga teachers engage in alternative physical exercise such as swimming, running, or surfing and rarely touch postural yoga. This is especially prevalent later in life through maturation on the path. This circumstance, while more uncommon in the West, shows that yoga isn't exclusively about asana for them. It is certainly a perspective to be curious about. Millions of people in India do not practice asana, yet so much of the philosophical teachings and general way of life in India is inextricably tied to yoga and related to the Vedic sciences. Recognizing this, we may uncover a clue to our solidarity and progress as a global community of yoga practitioners.

Should anyone feel the call to pursue a life guided by yoga, one that aims to integrate the teachings and practices, surely an attempt to understand its history would be an ethical place to start. This entire section serves only as a bird's-eye view of what we know so far, but it does begin to indicate a cultural context for the development of yoga within India. Whether you are a student or also a teacher of yoga, it is undeniable that understanding the customs and heritage of the country ensures that our individual application of yoga is far more virtuous. As archaeologists and academics continue their diligent efforts in research, more connections and clarifications will be brought to light over the years to come. While there are still missing links and, on the surface, there are teachings that seem contradictory to one another, one key component of yoga that is certain is that the path and practices are intended to take us inward. Over time, yoga is designed to take us from exclusively outer identification, alchemically inward through the most subtle layers of the self, and then beyond.

CONTEMPLATIONS

What is yoga? How would I define and describe yoga to another person?

What are the origins of the yoga that I personally practice?

How can I respectfully represent and uphold the roots of yoga?

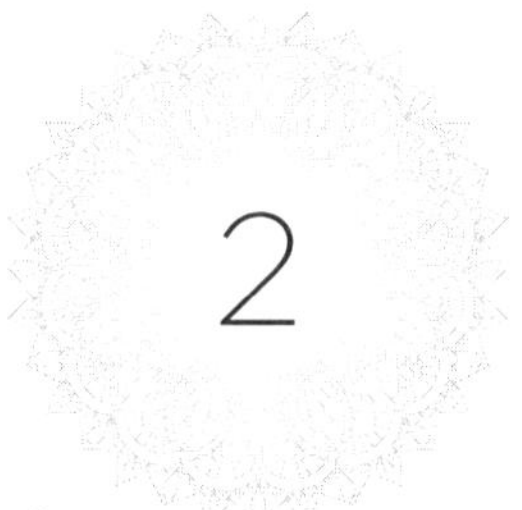

YOGIC ANATOMY

According to yogic thought, the human body is a microcosmic universe and also a part of the macrocosmic universe itself. The edges of the visual body blend and dissolve into that which the human eye cannot see. Each body will, one day, go back to the earth. Do we truly understand the origin of each individual body? Could it be that it starts as a tiny seed within our mother, and within her mother, tracing our physical manifestation back through time? Where does our body truly begin and end? What is this vessel carrying or containing, beyond its visible anatomical structure? If one's body is part of the greater universe, then does everything around oneself contain the same fundamental fabric as the body does, and at all times? If one were to transcend this physical body and its perceived limits, what would happen to that physical container? Then, was the body truly contained in the first place? Is the separate, individual self a reality or a grand illusion?

With deeper and continued inquiry, superficial conundrums begin to fade away. Yoga can teach us to constantly experience an awe toward life, both the physical and subtle. An intimate exploration of the subtle body taps us into a remarkable understanding of how we are both of the world and, simultaneously, beyond it.

Taking a pilgrimage into the body, through refined and consistent techniques, allows us the insight to directly experience the various points of our own temple. This includes working with various plexuses—the *marmas*, the chakras, the granthis—and an entire web of interconnectedness. Each sacred site within the subtle body holds its own value and *shakti* (energy). Even in the most generic way, we can look to the chakra system and the ornamental symbology of the body to barely grasp the value of knowing ourselves to be an expression of the holiest and most divine aspect of nature and existence itself. This contemplation of our inner temple is inclusive of both the manifest and unmanifest reality.

Turning briefly to Ayurvedic wisdom, consider when we mindfully prepare the most nourishing food for ourselves, as if it were an offering for a *puja* within our own temple. We go on to eat with incredible attentiveness and receive the gift of fuel for the body and mind. With this level of awareness and intention, we receive deep nourishment like *prasad* (pruh-SAH-d) that is offered then received back, as we might experience at a temple in India. The meal has transformed into nectar. For many of us, our modern lifestyle drives us into disconnection from this personal temple and inner ritual, resulting in consuming our meals in a rushed and thoughtless manner.

Numerous teachings guide us to view the body as a temple, something integral to living yoga, but not merely in an external, superficial way. The path of yoga can call us to seek out the richness of the vessel we are inhabiting, that is, to go within and explore the subtle terrain. If we utilize the practice for inward evolution and not outward gain, yoga warmly invites us to withdraw and rest within the quietude of our residence.

Prana

As with all Sanskrit words, context is important. There are always multiple translations of any given word within this sacred and classical language. For the purpose of this entire section, grasping the concept of prana is vital (no pun intended). Prana is the energy or force of life that animates any living thing. Prana fuels and sustains us, just as the concept of *ch'i* or *qi* within Traditional Chinese medicine. This life energy governs biological processes and more specifically the breath.

The word *prana* also implies air, especially concerning its various directions of movement, such as that of *prana vayu* versus *apana* (ap-AH-nuh) *vayu*. It is connected to the breath, but it is not exclusively the breath itself. Prana is not only inherently within each animate being, but it is also received through food, water, sunshine, and the air we inhale. Naturally, the quality of prana affects the quality of life. Within the body, prana is believed to move through pathways called *nadis*, much like the concept of meridians in Traditional Chinese Medicine. In both yoga and Ayurveda, it is taught that we must keep efficient circulation of prana throughout the body for optimal physical and mental health. So, in a practical sense, the accurate and constructive mobilization of prana within the body through yogic techniques can be attributed to greater health, healing, and the reduction of disease. Prana is one of the crucial elements that brings greater potency and vigor into daily life, and it thereby contributes to our overall long-term vitality and radiance. The primary direction for working with prana within the context of yoga is to amplify the results of our physical practice and eventually move toward the illumination of enlightenment.

Sharira Traya

A complete yoga practice (*sarvanga sadhana*) will ideally consider the *sharira traya*. *Traya* is a Sanskrit word that means "threefold," "three divisions," "triple," "three parts," "three kinds," or simply "three." It can also be said as *trayam* or *treya*. *Sharira* (sha-REE-ruh) is a Sanskrit word meaning, in this context, "body." Another relevant word for body, used interchangeably, is *deha*. The sharira traya represents the three bodies of each individual person. Ideally, any yoga practice, or sadhana, considers its impact on and relationship with these layers of the self. This yogic journey inward is a progressive interiorization.

Sthula sharira is the most tangible aspect of the individual self—the gross or physical body. It is that part of the individual self that is composed of the five elements: *bhumi* (earth), *prana* (air), *agni* (fire), *jala* (water), and *akasha* (ether). This outer body is our primary instrument to engage with the world. It reflects our accumulation of karmas and is the tool by which we create new karmas. The sthula sharira is our mortal body, and therefore our physiology that we experience during our conscious state. It is ever-changing yet impermanent, or finite. This body is bound by the laws of prakriti—that which is manifest. It is all that we can see and sense of ourselves in the waking state. At this level, we work to release physical rigidity and tension that is both consciously and unconsciously held throughout the body. Sthula sharira, regarding our consciousness, relates to our waking state.

Sukshma sharira is a more subtle aspect of the individual self. It is the pranic body and that which thereby animates the previous sthula sharira. Sometimes called the astral body, this subtle layer of self relates to the actions of the five pranas, or vayus. These are the five directions or functions of prana in the body (*prana*, *apana*, *samana*, *udana*, and *vyana*). When we die, the subtle body perishes alongside the gross body.

This subtle body is in relationship with the organs of action and the organs of the senses. It is associated with the thoughts and motivations that drive our actions in the world through the physical body. Hence the sukshma sharira reflects the part of the mind called *manas*. Manas is the aspect of the mind that is in direct relationship to the senses and therefore how we interact with the world around us. This layer also reflects the *buddhi*, the discerning aspect of the mind, alongside memory as *smriti* and the ego (or I-ness) as *ahamkara*. It is within the sukshma sharira that we begin to resolve the subconscious, conditioned blockages within both prana and the mind. It is associated with the state of dreaming and the subconscious.

Karana sharira, the causal body, is beyond the gross tangible self, the subtle anatomical structures, and the mind. As the most subtle and hidden aspect of the self, it is here we dance on the edge of dissolution into the universal consciousness, where any awareness of the individual self ceases to exist. This deepest layer is where we house the most engrained habits, karma, and samskaras that drive our life trajectory. Through consistent yoga practices that work with the subtle yogic anatomy and pranic body, given they are interrelated with this causal body, obstructions can potentially be cleared. We can then begin to experience a heightened awareness of our truest essence and state.

Associated with dreamless sleep or the unconscious, this is a layer of self that we can barely contemplate an experience of, as it blurs the boundaries of time and space. The causal body is the aspect of the individual that is believed to be eternal. It is the seed form of an individual. Only within the most supreme meditative states can we consider accessing the karana sharira. One of the aims of yoga is to transcend all these perceived layers of the individual self and experience a merging with the ultimate reality.

Pancha Kosha

Related to the previous traya sharira, the *pancha* (five) *kosha* are very similar in that they give us a framework to understand the journey through the layers of the self, from the gross to the most subtle. Derived from the *Taittiriya Upanishad*, and therefore also taught within Vedanta philosophy, the five sheaths of the "body" are like lampshades that progressively cover the light within us. As we move from the outer to the inner, each of the layers has less and less *tamas* within. The five koshas are also mentioned and utilized within the Hatha yoga tradition. These koshas are similar to, but very evidently not the same as, the five layers of consciousness taught in Tantra. We will circle back to these for an interesting comparison at the end of this section.

Annamaya kosha is the outer, most physical layer of the koshas, much like the sthula sharira. *Anna*, translated from Sanskrit, most commonly means "food." Just as the goddess Annapurna is associated with food, sustenance, and nourishment, this layer is about the gross body and what we take in. When tending to the annamaya kosha, the goal is to nurture the body so we can enjoy our external lives. As a result, this helps us to go inward without the body being any hindrance.

This sheath corresponds to our physical movements and sensory experience interacting with the world. It emphasizes the understanding that whatever we consume directly impacts our level of wellness. Hence our diet and lifestyle choices are paramount to the vitality of the annamaya kosha. Weaving in an Ayurvedic perspective, both the quality and quantity of food are valuable considerations, as each directly impacts the state of one's *jathara agni*, or the primary digestive fire. A digestive system that is out of balance can result in poor sleep, poor skin health, and more. Postural yoga is an important tool to work with this outer sheath, given that it supports the health of all the organs and systems of the worldly, mortal body, as are the cleansing shatkriya techniques found in Hatha yoga. Receiving regular sunlight is another common means of bringing the annamaya kosha into a harmonious state.

Pranamaya kosha is regarded as the subtle or pranic body. It is the sheath that is composed of our vital energy. Like the annamaya kosha, it is fueled by breath, sunlight, and high-quality plant foods. This kosha can be likened to an organizational field, one that holds the material body together. Consider the previous description of prana and its application here. It is this pranic energy that supports the optimal function of respiration, circulation, and digestion, thereby supporting various bodily functions. The constructive movement or circulation of prana indicates the health of this sheath. Undeniably, the breath is the primary carrier of prana within the body, hence pranayama is the most straightforward, practical way to work with this layer of oneself. Pranamaya kosha is the bridge between the body and mind, therefore any mental or emotional disturbances can be attributed to blockages within this sheath. In terms of the most commonplace aspects of the yogic subtle anatomy, it is here that we associate the nadis and chakras, for example.

Manomaya kosha is the mind-body (or mental layer) of the self, which comprises our passing thoughts, emotions, perceptions, and cognitive processes. These mental afflictions arise within us like undercurrents, or otherwise waves in the ocean. The term *manomaya* pulls from the Sanskrit word *manas*, meaning "mind." Considering the constant inner dialogue that impacts our perception of reality, this sheath often appears to have a strong hold on us. The manomaya kosha filters the sensory input received via the sense organs. In turn, our reactions and behavior within the world are commonly driven by this aspect of the self. It could be said that the manomaya kosha is the location where the formation and manifestation of both our samskaras and vasanas occur. Each of these drive attachments and the pursuit of desires within the world. This kosha is also the root of the five kleshas, or mental causes of suffering. These concepts will be expanded upon later in this chapter. Practices that serve the manomaya kosha are those that promote pratyahara, or sensory withdrawal. Self-inquiry and meditation are crucial. Recitation of Vedic mantras would also be an aid to this mental sheath.

Vijnanamaya kosha, the fourth layer, represents the discernment and intelligence that is underneath, or beyond, the thinking aspect of the mind. It relates to our intuition and inherent wisdom. This sheath guides our ethical and moral choices from a higher knowledge via critical thinking, reason, direct experience, and emotional equanimity. It relates to deep spiritual inquiry and practice and plays a significant role in moving toward Self-realization. The Sanskrit word *vijnana* translates to "recognizing," "intelligence," "discernment," and "proficiency." Accessing this deeper layer of self requires a consistent, steady, and balanced state of the three prior koshas. It is only through diligent practice, time, experience, and maturation that we can reach the potential of the vijnanamaya kosha. It is here we uncover the supreme higher states of yoga that are only accessed through meditation.

Anandamaya kosha is the final, innermost layer of the self. *Ananda* is a Sanskrit word most frequently translated as "bliss." Here we go entirely beyond the mind and into a state of simply being, one that could be characterized by boundless bliss, Self-remembrance, or Self-realization. To reside in this state, where we can potentially experience the dissolution of all ego, mental activity, and all desires, is regarded as an ultimate goal of yoga. Anandamaya kosha offers an experience that is beyond the ordinary realm, beyond individual identification. Here we uncover a seemingly eternal essence of each person and our interconnectedness with all of creation.

The differing Tantrik perspective on the layers of self is equally valuable, despite being much lesser known. A framework that is emphasized specifically within the Non-Dual Shaiva Tantra (NST) tradition, the five layers are sometimes taught with a preliminary sixth outer layer called *vastu* (vas-tu). Not to be confused with the Indian system of sacred design and architecture also called Vastu (VAH-stu), this sixth layer relates to material possessions and wealth, the things we surround ourselves with. Vastu points to the things we own (that often own *us*!). The Sanskrit word translates to "object," "article," "substance of anything," "contents," "goods," "wealth," "property," and more.

Much the same as annamaya kosha, the next layer, which is the first main outer layer in the Tantrik system, is *deha*, or body. This layer is associated with the physical body that will eventually age and die. From here, the Vedantic koshas and the NST layers of the self diverge. After the layer of physicality, we learn of *chitta*, or the heart-mind. The mental thoughts and emotions are placed between the physical and pranic body, given they're directly connected to the senses. This layer of chitta

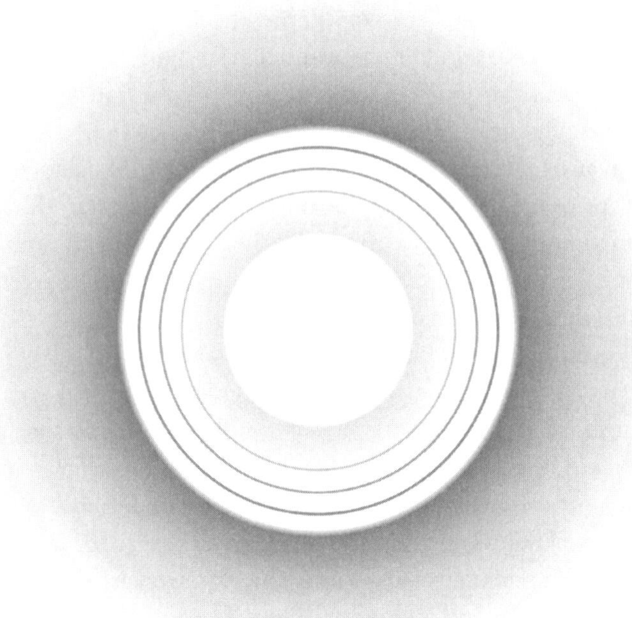

FIGURE 1. The panca koshas

is reflected in the suffering we experience from not seeing things as they truly are. It is here that we repeat thoughts and reactions until they become engrained habits that impact the way we physically and mentally engage in the world. The sense organs are the bridge between the physical body and the mind. Hence it makes sense that they are intimately side by side in this systematic approach to the self.

Seen as more subtle than our mental afflictions is the pranic body. Prana has no boundaries and connects us to all living animate beings. It is where we begin to transcend our individuality. Prana permeates the layers of chitta and deha, given it is impacted by food, water, sunlight, and air. Reciprocally, the quality of prana, that is, whether it is depleted or bountiful, will impact the mind and the body. However, prana is regarded as far more fundamental to our core existence. Like the pranamaya kosha, this pranic layer relates to the five vayus (winds), which we will explore further in the following section.

More subtle again is the next layer, called *shunya*. This Sanskrit word is translated as "void," "empty," "non-entity," and "vacuum." It is a state of self that is most commonly accessed through deep stillness, meditation, and dreamless sleep. It is regarded as the profoundly peaceful state of self, beyond identification with the outer world. Many who have a transcendent experience between the inner and outer realities may describe it as witnessing something all-pervasive.

Last, we come to the core, *chit*. This omnipresent center of our being pervades all layers of self. It is virtually impossible to describe or grasp, because it is beyond anything objective. It is the pulsating existence of everything within each of us. It is the Supreme Reality and pure consciousness that powers everything we perceive. Although it is described as the core, it exists everywhere, in everything. Understanding this reality of our true nature is at the heart of Tantrik teachings. When we come to the deep realization that everything is divinity vibrating into manifestation at all times, our identity shifts, and we see everything as sacred. By plugging into this core, we experience a freedom that offers us the capacity to embrace the manifest reality with joy, curiosity, and reverence. Here we move from the depths of meditative transcendence, expanding back outward to a new level of embodied wholeness.

Vayu

Revered across Hindu, Jain, and Buddhist scripture is the god of wind and breath, Vayu (VAH-yu). He is the father of the well-known devotional and loyal monkey god, Hanuman. Vayu is one of several guardians of the directions called Dikpala (dik-PAH-la). In this case, he is the deity associated with the North-West direction. We can learn more about the deity Vayu through various shastras such as the Rigveda, the Upanishads, and the Mahabharata. Most significantly, Vayu is responsible for carrying the breath of life and is particularly affiliated with the vital life force known as *prana vayu*.

The word *vayu* is associated with three *doshas* of Ayurveda, namely the *vata* (vah-ta) dosha. One Sanskrit translation of the word *vayu* is "air," and vata comprises the air and space elements. Uncovering the meaning of the vayus brings us closer to understanding the animation of our human existence, of our essential life force. Within the context of yogic anatomy, aside from referring to the breath, vayu represents the vital air, or the five winds. This includes their directions and actions within the subtle body. These five vayus are *prana vayu*, *apana vayu*, *samana vayu*, *udana vayu*, and *vyana vayu*. These vayus are *upadoshas*; they are subfunctions of the vata dosha. Each serves to move the prana in a certain manner. Understanding these five vayus helps us to have a more intimate relationship with vata, which is essential for us in our stimulated and fast-paced society. The more physical aspects of a yoga practice, such as asana, bandha, mudra, and pranayama, influence all five vayus and aid in promoting the optimal movement of each. In turn, the five vayus animate physical and mental functions due to and through the air quality. This again relates to vata, which governs all aspects of movement. Mention of the five vayus is found mainly across Hatha texts and in the Yoga Upanishads.

Prana vayu is associated with right-nostril breathing, given its connection to *pingala nadi*. It energizes, revitalizes, and internalizes. It is an inward force; hence it has a relationship to inhalations. It is additionally related to the upward force of prana, unless the action is reversed through the process of merging with apana vayu, thereby igniting kundalini. Prana vayu is seated in the *hrdayam* (spiritual heart center) and also in the head. Working with prana vayu aims to build and recharge our energy. Specific techniques include the engagement of asanas that involve mostly backbends (both active and restorative), some lateral postures, *uddiyana* (uddi-YAH-na) bandha, pranayama that emphasizes right-nostril breathing, and *antara kumbhaka*, the breath retention after an *inhalation*.

Apana vayu is related to a descending or downward-moving action of prana. It governs elimination, menstruation, childbirth, and the reproductive and urinary systems. It relates to the lower abdomen, organs of elimination, and the pelvic floor, for men and women. Apana vayu relates to left-nostril breathing, activating *ida nadi*, which grounds us. It promotes steadiness of body and mind. Working with apana vayu requires engagement of forward-folding asanas, mulabandha, and pranayama that emphasizes both left-nostril breathing and also *bahya kumbhaka*, breath retention after an *exhalation*. The activation of kundalini is generally due to the merging of apana and prana vayu within the navel center, occurring when each has reversed its direction to unite with the other. We will decode this a little more in the next section.

Samana vayu assumes an assimilating action of prana. It is essential for digestion, of both the physical and mental kind. The Sanskrit root word *sama* can be translated as "equal," "moderate," "good," "whole," "constant," "uniform," or "balanced." Samana vayu is the vital wind that circulates around the navel area and on the head at the hair whorl. Physically, it is mostly related to the stomach and intestinal tract. In addition, it is associated with how we assimilate our mental and emotional afflictions alongside the impressions we take in, such as those that come through conversation or the media. It also has a relationship to the eyes and sense of sight. In Ayurveda, samana vayu is considered to impact the digestive fire directly. This includes the *jathara* and *bhuta* agnis. Jathara agni is the more physical, commonplace digestive function. Bhuta agni is the subtle and elemental digestion of food and nutrients. Engaging yoga postures that twist and rotate the spine as well as *mayurasana*, one of the earliest nonseated asanas, stimulating kriyas such as *kapalabhati* (ka-PAH-la-BHAH-tee), and consuming a *sattvic* diet are all ways to tend to samana vayu in an accessible way.

Udana vayu relates to the ascending force of prana. In the context of the five vayus, the Sanskrit word *udana* implies breathing upward, or the vital air within the throat that moves upward. It is particularly associated with our speech and verbal expression. Outwardly, udana vayu is reflected in our decision-making, our creativity, and our capacity for enthusiasm toward life in general. Udana vayu is centered within the throat and also the crown of the head, the third eye, and the heart. It is udana vayu that aids in the ascension of kundalini once prana and apana have united. In terms of asanas, a steady inversion is useful in working with this vayu. This is not limited to the typical inversions such as headstand; it includes anything elevating the hips over the heart and head, like *adho mukha shvanasana* (downward-facing dog posture). Working with the three major bandhas—mulabandha, uddiyana, and jalandhara—is also useful, as is *nauli kriya* (the isolation and churning of the abdominal muscles). When inverting the body, we are not only reversing gravity on the physical body, but we are also working to retain the flow of *amrita*. Amrita, sometimes also called *soma*, is the metaphysical and divine nectar of immortality located in the head. It is what is said to bestow a practitioner with eternal life through spiritual awakening.

Vyana vayu is the diffusing and circulating action of prana within the subtle body. It distributes and expands, integrating all of the vayus. We could liken it in its entirety to a bubble or aura that pervades and surrounds the entire body. Vyana promotes a harmonious union of the vayus together through its integrative nature. The Sanskrit word *vyana* is commonly translated as "circulate" or "pervade." Both reflect the essence of the vayu well. We could liken vyana vayu to a subtle version of the physical circulatory system. It functions throughout the entire body, including all of the *indriyas*, which are the sense and motor organs. Most lineages loosely teach that this vayu has no specific seat or organ within the body, but some believe it is anchored in the hrdayam and expands outward from there. While all movement in general is excellent for supporting vyana vayu, lateral opening poses are regarded as ideal. Also beneficial are those that circulate awareness toward the outer limbs and encourage movement of the lymphatic system. All pranayama serves vyana vayu. Any body or breath practices that act like a pump can be advantageous if performed safely with the stability of apana vayu.

There is a heavy emphasis in modern yoga on physical alignment and Western anatomy and physiology. This attention on the outer practices, and therefore the outer layer of self, can take us only so far. It is certainly useful as an entry point for beginners to postural yoga or for the prevention of injury and recovery of the physical body. However, a maturing yoga practice brings attention to how we shape prana and thereby purposefully progress in our practice. It is worth noting here that there are ten vayus in total. The other five, the *nagadi vayus*, are less relevant to the yoga practice and relate to the function of the autonomic nervous system. They are *naga* (pronounced NAH-ga, this is the eructation reflex and the free intuitive movement of the body), *kurma* (the blinking of the eyelids), *krkara* (the sneezing reflex, hunger sensation, and belching), *devadatta* (yawning), and *dhanamjaya* (heart pulsations, sound movement throughout the body, and bodily decomposition after death).

Nadi

The word *nadi* is most often used in Sanskrit to indicate a tubular-shaped organ (such as veins and arteries), the stalk of a plant, the pulse, a unit of time (that is, twenty-four minutes), or in yoga, a subtle channel within the body. Across the numerous texts and traditions in India, the common consensus is that there are 72,000 of these subtle channels within the human body that originate from a *kanda* (bulb) located slightly below the *manipura* chakra. Much like the system of meridians in Traditional Chinese Medicine, it is thought that the nadis are pathways running throughout the body that conduct energy. These conduits of prana are believed to run between or through the chakras. They also conjoin in other plexus centers across the subtle body such as the marmas (vital energy points). The nadis are acknowledged across a range of texts such as the Yoga Upanishads, the Hatha Pradipika, the Tantras, and also throughout some Buddhist teachings.

Within Eastern and Western texts that mention these subtle channels, the general agreement is that there are three major, and therefore most important, nadis. These are *ida* (ee-DAH), *pingala* (pin-gal-AH), and *sushumna* (su-shum-NAH) nadi. In Tantrik Buddhism, or Vajrayana ("Diamond Vehicle"), the same three major nadis are named *lalana*, *rasana*, and *avadhuti*. Ida and pingala nadis are sometimes said to run along either side of the central channel. They are said to coil around the sushumna nadi, intersecting and crossing back and forth as they make their way upward. These places where the two repeatedly converge are understood to be the locations of the major chakras.

Ida nadi is located on the left, originating at the base of the torso and running up into the head, ending at the left nostril. The word *ida* translates to "comfort." Its qualities are cooling and calming, relating to the parasympathetic nervous system. Ida is associated with *chandra* (the moon), feminine yin energy, and the river Ganga, or Ganges. Ida is stimulated when we inhale, as it is naturally cooler than the exhalation. Lying down on one's right side is a simple way to open ida nadi.

Pingala nadi is located on the right side, originating at the base of the torso, running into the head and ending at the right nostril. The word *pingala* translates to "tawny," referring to an orange-brown color. Its qualities relate to warmth, vitality, and activity. It is in relationship with the sympathetic nervous system. Pingala is associated with *surya* (the sun), masculine yang energy, and the river Yamuna. Pingala is stimulated when we exhale, as it is naturally warmer than the inhalation. Lying down on one's left side is a simple way to open pingala nadi.

A crucial function of the yoga practice is to ensure any obstructions within these two nadis and the nadi system overall are removed. Techniques such as shatkriya, mudra, and pranayama are utilized to clear any energetic blockages. When they are understood correctly, the tools can be applied to both open and close certain nadis. This is specifically to promote the opening of sushumna nadi. Sushumna is said to have three layers. Within the third, most subtle layer, the chakras are created and located. Sushumna is also believed to have three directions of flow. These are *arohana* (upward), *avarohana* (downward), and *vajrini* (thrusting).

The goal with the three major nadis is to ultimately invigorate the dormant kundalini, which rests near the base of the spine (the exact location varies depending on the text), and to send it up sushumna nadi. Generally, the ideal time to work on moving prana into sushumna is around dawn and dusk. This is one of the reasons why the daily windows of *brahmamuhurta* (early morning, predawn hours) and *goraj muhurta* (evening hours) are so valuable in yogic traditions. In addition, the "door" to sushumna is open only when both nostrils are equally in balance, which may reflect why there is great emphasis on the accessible pranayama technique of *nadi shodhana*. Sushumna relates to fire and the river Saraswati (in addition, all nadis in the body are sometimes referred to as rivers). To activate kundalini, we merge apana and prana vayus at the navel to create the subtle sacred fire, sometimes called *rudrani.*

> Realizing that a man's body is like an electric battery, I reasoned that it could be recharged with energy through the direct agency of human will.[1]

Kundalini in its dormant state rests coiled at the base of the spine near the first and second chakras, *muladhara* and *svadhishthana*. At least, this is the most common belief, driven by the teachings of Hatha yoga. In her dwelling place, kundalini is likened to a serpent and thus ascribed a reptilian nature. Consider how serpents shed their skin to come forth renewed. In a similar light, our yoga practice requires us to strip away and shed old conditioning. *Kundalini shakti* (often called "serpentine power" as a metaphor) in a quiescent state requires advanced practices to rise.

Kundalini is revered as a divine feminine energy that pushes us toward transformation. Consider the nature of fire itself. Fire rises and transforms in the same manner that kundalini desires to purify us. When she rises, kundalini can become united with amrita, the divine nectar located in the head. This is a transcendental approach to working with kundalini. In her coiled springlike shape, she represents our *potential* of power. Kundalini is always awake, whether coiled or active. To demystify kundalini a little further, she is simply prana summoned via will through certain techniques. She is prana shakti, a state of one's own energy, not a kind of separate entity. This is much like the chakras, which we will come to. It is significant to highlight that activated, ascending, or descending kundalini does not amount to enlightenment. That is a very important disclosure.

Some of the practical applications that bring us closer to the arousal of kundalini include pranayama, mantra, and contemplation or meditation. Certain asanas, when utilized appropriately and when orienting us inward, can be useful too. The purpose of the postures is to prepare the body and mind for the process of working with prana, the nadis, and kundalini more intimately. In this context, ideally the main direction for any sincere practitioner should be to work with the ethereal system of nadis to remove subtle obstructions and move toward an increased vitality and life force. Any activation of kundalini is related to and could be regarded as similar to the experience of *shaktipat*. Shaktipat is most commonly considered to be a divine transmission from guru to disciple, via formal initiation, which can set in motion higher states of consciousness, either immediately or over time.

In closing, it must be said that the concept of kundalini has not been heavily studied in academia. Most Sanskrit sources that mention the word are yet to be translated and decoded. More significant to note is that any mention of kundalini here and within the Yoga Upanishads and the Tantras has no direct relationship to the modern practice of kundalini yoga made famous by Yogi Bhajan (born Harbhajan Singh Puri, 1929–2004). The word *kundalini* occurs possibly for the first time in written form in Tantrik texts of the seventh century C.E. Hence kundalini could be said to be a Tantrik doctrine that was later adopted within the subsequent Hatha tradition. It is also claimed that the first mention of the word is in the *Lalita Sahasranama*, found within the *Brahmanda Purana* (one of the oldest of the Puranas). Nonetheless, we will unravel and further expand upon kundalini in the next section due to its intimate relationship with the often-adulterated system of the chakras.

Chakra

With no intention to denigrate what most people understand the chakras to be, it is essential to highlight that the common Western interpretation is vastly different from that of the East—and the Indic philosophical systems specifically. The reality is that the chakras were adapted and innovated upon when they were translated to a Western audience roughly 150 years ago. This was due to the influence of multiple people and organizations. The most significant was the Theosophical Society and the well-known psychologist Carl Jung, who played a key role in the evolution of the chakra system as it is widely known today. Over the decades, New Age writers, energy healers, clairvoyants, and esotericists have been captivated by the concept of chakras and have contributed to ongoing modifications. The subtle and esoteric information surrounding the chakras in India was therefore transmuted by a Western perspective and bias when it was brought to the rest of the world. This is what resulted in the rainbow chakra system we commonly see plastered in books and across posters and paired with aromatherapy oils and crystals at annual spirituality expos. This modern framework became somewhat standardized into a six-plus-one structure: the "one" being *sahasrara*, the "crown" chakra.

The Sanskrit word *chakra* (correctly pronounced cha-kr, not shah-krah) has several translations. Most relevant would be "wheel," "whirlpool," "circle," and "cycle." There are numerous variations in the chakra system within India. Some texts and traditions reference only one chakra. Some refer to four, five, seven, nine, and even fifteen or more chakras. Others mention none at all. These chakras are sites where nadis converge together. While we see reference to colors associated with the chakras in Indian philosophy, it is *not* a rainbow system. In fact, traditionally each major chakra has two or more colors. In contrast, the Western approach designates one specific color to each chakra, resulting in the now-popularized rainbow order.

Within India, synonyms for the word *chakra* are used interchangeably—for example, *adhara*, *sthana*, *lakshya*, and *padma*. This alone begins to highlight how the Indian chakra system is far more esoteric and nuanced than that of the Western world, which was wildly altered and eventually commodified. A significant book that appears to have somewhat synthesized the Eastern application of the chakra system is the *Shat-Chakra-Nirupana* by Swami Purnananda. The date of this work is hard to pin down, but it is probably a sixteenth-century text, very likely from 1577. It teaches of the six major chakra centers, which are to be used in meditation specifically. The Sanskrit word *shaṭ* means "six." *Nirupana* means "investigation," "examination," "sight," "form," or "shape."

Alas, little is known about Swami Purnananda. It is suggested that he was a Bengali yogi and a Tantrika. Nonetheless, the *Shat-Chakra-Nirupana* was translated and published within *The Serpent Power*, an exposition of Tantra published in 1919 by Arthur Avalon. Arthur Avalon was the pseudonym of Sir John Woodroffe. Woodroffe (1865–1936) was a British judge on the high court of Calcutta (now Kolkata), India. He was also a student of Tantra. *The Serpent Power* was the first time a concise presentation of the Eastern chakra framework was brought to the West. However, the information in the text is a notable catalyst for codifying the six-plus-one system that has become famous in the past several decades. Therefore, the book could be considered a pivotal turning point, marking the shift in development between the Eastern and Western understanding of the chakras.

Particularly within, but not limited to, the Tantrik traditions, the chakras were always intended to be visualized as focal points in meditation. They are believed to be conceptual structures present in the subtle body, within the pranayama kosha or the sukshma sharira. There may also be structures in the physical body that indicate an *association* with the chakras and where they are concentrated. However, these are phenomenological and strictly part of the subtle anatomy. It could be suggested that the chakras do not exist until they are created through the mind, pending the particular practice one is performing. While they were engaged during meditation in Tantrik traditions, it would be more appropriate to say that they were to be "installed" or "placed" in certain locations throughout the body based on the goal of the practice. The technique of placing the chakras in a focused location during meditation was a means to establishing a mantra or deity within the chosen site. This place-holding technique is called *nyasa* (ny-AH-sa). *Nyasa* translates from Sanskrit to "fixing," "applying," "inserting," "impressing," "placing," or "putting down." It is a technique used across the entire body in different contexts, such as during puja.

In terms of the traditional composition of the chakras, aside from the use of two or more colors, there are other cardinal features. These include the following:

Association with a plane or realm of existence, called a *loka*, from gross to most subtle (there are believed to be seven lokas)

Individual sounds of the Sanskrit alphabet designated on each petal on any chakra

A yantra (in this context, a simple symbol representing an element associated with the chakra)

A *bija* (a seed syllable that can be used visually and audibly)

A *vahana* (an animal that acts as a carrier for the particular bija and the element)

A representation of a *devata* with *devi* (deities that correlate with Shiva and Shakti)

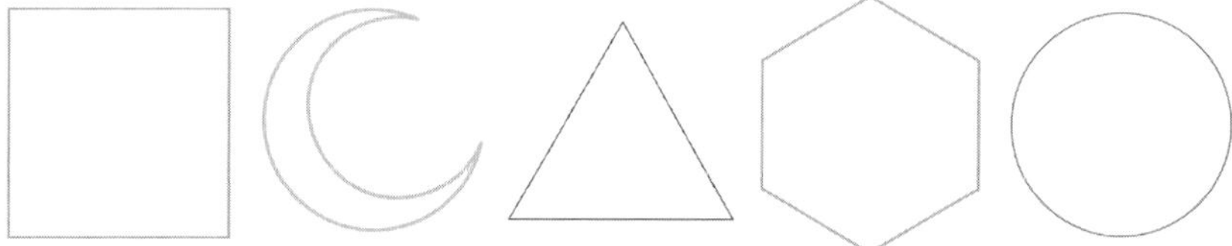

FIGURE 2. The pancha mahabhuta (five element) yantra symbols that are sometimes used with a corresponding chakra

The seed mantras used are sometimes said to be LAAM, VAAM, RAAM, YAAM, and HAAM. Alternatively, we can also learn of HRAAM, HREEM, HROOM, HRAIM, and HRAUM, which are linked to kundalini. Either way, the bija mantras are in direct relationship to the element being installed in a chakra. This means that, contrary to common belief, a bija mantra is not affiliated exclusively with one set chakra. The seed mantra belongs to the *element*, and the Tantrik approach is that any element can be installed across any chakra, again according to the purpose of the practice. In Tantra, the chakras have always been viewed as both prescriptive and customizable, within the framework of the features just listed.

Some traditions suggest that most of the major chakras reside within the subtlest layer of sushumna nadi. In this case, we can truly access the chakras only when we can successfully and steadily arouse sushumna nadi. This means that the chakras are pierced when kundalini ascends to her "final" destination, the sahasrara chakra, and also when she descends back down through the central channel. This destination of the crown chakra is a perspective more so of the Hatha tradition, for those who wish to transcend the body. It is indicated across various Tantrik sources that kundalini may be also activated at the heart, and that kundalini may both ascend and descend to unite in the heart (similar to the action of apana and prana vayu merging). There are Tantrik teachings that indicate a belief that kundalini may reside near the heart. Others suggest she rests coiled near the navel. This is in contrast, again, to the more common idea in Hatha yoga that kundalini is placed near the lower spine, within the pelvis.

In addition, the polymath and Kashmir philosopher Abhinavagupta (950–1016 C.E.) taught of the three kundalinis—a kundalini triad. They are *para-kundalini* near the crown (also called *urdhva-kundalini*), *kula-kundalini* at the heart (sometimes also called *chit-kundalini*), and *prana-kundalini* near the base (also called *adha-kundalini*). This concept of the three kundalinis has greater relevance for those who wish to become fully enlivened in their human form as a means to embracing life while simultaneously moving toward higher states. It is certainly a more Tantrik line of thought. It is an approach that encourages a descent of the upper kundalini as a means to ensure embodiment of our human form and existence. Classical Tantra also holds the idea that kundalini is therefore also the source of the three primary shaktis (*iccha*, *jnana*, and *kriya* shaktis) and is a phonemic power, meaning that she is the source of the entire Sanskrit alphabet. Evidently, kundalini is a vast and mysterious subject.

Similar in some sense to the chakras—as locations within the subtle body that require deliberate attention—are the three primary granthis. The Sanskrit word *granthi* most commonly translates to "a knot." The granthis are psychic knots that are believed to bind us on the path to Self-realization. They are a barrier to knowing reality, or that which is beyond the individual self. They hold us in our mental patterns and resistance, an idea that we will unpack in the following section, which focuses on the mind. The three major knots are *brahmagranthi, vishnugranthi,* and *rudragranthi.* According to some schools and traditions of both yoga and Tantra, there are more than three granthis. These additional secondary granthis reflect the complexity of human conditioning, psychology, and karma.

Brahmagranthi is situated around the base of the spine, between the muladhara and svadhishthana chakras. It relates to attachment associated with material security, survival, and the primitive brain. It is reflected in a fear of change, possessiveness, and a lack of groundedness.

Vishnugranthi is located near the manipura and *anahata* chakras. It is connected to our sense of identity, power, and self-worth. It relates to the attachment associated with power, possessions, and manipulation that impede and dominate spiritual growth. We can see it related to the inability to maintain or develop meaningful relationships and connections with others.

Rudragranthi is located near or within the head, more commonly around the *ajna* chakra, but it can be situated between the anahata and ajna chakras. Also called the *mayagranthi,* it relates to spiritual awareness, the intellect, and a sense of unity with others. Its presence can be reflected in intellectual arrogance, resentment toward others when performing service, or spiritual superiority.

Numerous texts mention the granthis, such as the Tantras, Yoga Upanishads, Bhagavad Gita, Yoga Vasishtha, and multiple Hatha works. The granthis are responsible for blocking the effective movement of prana through sushumna nadi. Generally, like working with the chakras, the activation and directing of kundalini is the main technique used to pierce and dissolve the three granthis. They could be likened to the firm base of a flower bud. Once pierced, the flower is free to bloom, metaphorically speaking. In a practical sense, aside from pranayama and *kumbhaka* (breath retention), various mudras and bandhas are the key tools for working successfully with the granthis. Very specific mantras are also said to have the potential to disintegrate the rudragranthi. Like a needle (*suchi*), the sound (*nada*)—when resonated correctly—penetrates the knot, freeing upper kundalini energy.

Another association with the chakras is the several *marmani* (mar-MAH-nee) throughout the physical body. Marmanis (more commonly called *marma*) are the vital energy points that concentrate along intersections of the nadis, which only exist when prana is flowing properly through any location. *Marma cikitsa*, or marma therapy, is highly regarded within Ayurveda and the South Indian martial art tradition *kalaripayat*. When a marma site is injured, it can block the associated nadi and create pranic congestion or obstruction.

The marmas could be likened to a bridge between the physical and subtle body. They are certain locations all over the body that are very much like acupressure points. However, the marmas should not be confused with Chinese acupuncture sites, despite the belief that acupuncture has origins tied directly to Ayurveda. When manipulated and palpated, the *marmasthana* (meaning "vital or vulnerable place") can impact the physical, subtle, and mental bodies. This practice is a tool to remove obstructions and improve the flow of prana. Palpation of the marmas is a diagnostic method specifically for those qualified in Ayurvedic bodywork and massage. Similarly, yoga postures can be used to gently tend to the various marmas, governing the interchange of information between the outer and inner or the physical and subtle.

Finally, another subtle body concept is that of the three *bindus*. This pertains specifically and exclusively to Tantrik thought (although the word *bindu* has many meanings and uses across numerous traditions). The Sanskrit word translates most commonly to "drop," "dot," or "point." These three Tantrik bindus are located within the abdominal, heart, and head areas, and have single color associations. The bindus are sometimes regarded as so subtle that they are considered to be a part of the *causal* body. Importantly, they are not to be confused with the granthis, although the bindus do correspond to the three knots.

In Eastern thought, unlike in the West, the chakras do *not* need to be balanced nor healed as such. Indian traditions appear to agree that the purpose of working with the chakras is to ultimately pierce, dissolve, and transcend them. Hence it is our mental limitations that restrict us from accessing and harnessing these centers. Historically, through the practice of yoga and Tantra, the chakras have served a purpose distinctly different from the modern Western application. Lord Krishna's flute (the bansuri) has six holes that represent the main chakras. As he plays his flute, the air blowing through symbolizes prana moving through the sushumna, piercing all the nadis and merging into higher consciousness.

Hence, in the stories of Krishna's pastimes, all who hear Krishna's flute are entranced and experience a yearning to be closer to the Supreme. This is a beautiful reflection of the deeper teachings that pertain to the subtle anatomy in the much older Eastern traditions. All the additional correspondences to the chakras, such as aromas, gemstones, minerals, totem animals, tarot, and even psychological states of emotion, are influenced by Western alternative healing practices; they are not found in any Sanskrit or Indic source.

Mapping the Mind

The organ of the brain is the physical site of our mental emotions and afflictions. As we cannot tangibly see our thoughts, let alone consciousness itself, we will explore the various subtle components of the mind and how they influence our path and practice of yoga. After all, the mental and emotional nature of the individual self is a part of the sukshma sharira. All the components of the mind in their unity are considered to be *antahkarana*—the totality of the human psyche. A commonly known term is the Sanskrit word *chitta*—not to be confused with *chit*, a term sometimes used to imply unconditioned consciousness or the Supreme Reality. Chitta usually refers to the collective field of the mind. It is likened to a blank canvas or a movie screen. Chitta includes the following aspects of the mind and is also the storehouse of our memories and samskaras (latent mental impressions of acts performed by the body or mind during a former state of existence). At least, this is the perspective that has been distilled from Patanjali's Yoga Sutras.

Through further exploration of yogic teachings, such as those of Samkhya philosophy, we learn of the various facets of the mind in greater depth. A system of *tattvas*, meaning "principles" or "truths," is taught within Samkhya philosophy (in which there are twenty-five tattvas) and also Kashmir Shaivism (in which there are eleven additional tattvas, thereby totaling thirty-six). Each system of tattvas includes three core components of the mind, which we will expand upon here. They are manas, ahamkara, and buddhi.

Manas is the thinking, recording, and processing mind. It is the most direct aspect of the mind, receiving all impressions through the five *jnanendriya*, the organs of sense perception, which relate to the five elements. These are the nose (earth), tongue (water), eyes (fire), skin (air), and ears (space). Therefore, manas is the faculty responsible for subconscious sense synthesizing and processing. As a result, it also has a reciprocal action whereby the mental intentions we formulate then dictate how we express ourselves through our sense and motor organs. This instrument of conscious thinking relates to both objectivity (via the organization of sensory input) and subjectivity (our emotions). It is the aspect of us that is tempted to entertain fears and doubts, for example, and loves to gather information.

Manas has an outward projection and, due to the information overload and fast-paced nature of modern society, it often needs to be tamed and made stable. Too many people give themselves over to the pleasures of the senses, in some cases developing addictions. As a result, we can fall entirely under the control of the external world and lose our innate sense of self. Manas can be infatuated with pleasure and have a strong aversion to pain. It is the aspect of the mind that most of us encounter when beginning a consistent meditation practice. Manas, in a balanced state, cultivates self-discipline, devotion, willpower, control of the senses, and steady concentration.

Ahamkara relates to the part of the mind that strongly identifies with the individual self and a sense of "mine." It is an aspect that creates labels around who we believe we are, such as what we look like, and associations with outer qualities, objects, or circumstances. It sees everything as subject and object. Because of this, it synthesizes the experiences acquired via manas and absorbs them into its constructed sense of self. Ahamkara reinforces the egoic identity and is the owner of all experiences.

Of course, the ego is required to function and operate within the human realm. It aids in socialization and differentiates us from other aspects of the surrounding external world. However, it is imperative that, as we aim to progress on the path of yoga, we witness the ego as it creates division daily through subjectivity and bias. It is what drives pride and delusional self-image. It is self-conscious by nature and most often leads to suffering. Ahamkara is our fictional narrative, with ourself as the main character. (Similar to ahamkara is the concept of *asmita*. Asmita is also translated to "egoism" and is a related concept. However, the nuance here is that asmita is mostly regarded as more subtle and refers to the fundamental awareness of one's individual existence. It is a little more neutral and is a state in which we consciously question our limited identity.) Ahamkara, in its positive state and purified, cultivates self-inquiry, right association, compassion, and spiritual aspiration. On this level, ahamkara can help us experience ourselves in all other things and, in turn, also see all things as within.

Buddhi is considered to be the most valuable mental faculty concerning spiritual progress. The Sanskrit word *buddhi*, within the context of Samkhya philosophy, means "intellect." However it also generally translates to "apprehension," "reasonable view," "right opinion," "presence of mind," "comprehension," and the "power of retaining discernment." Buddhi reflects a high level of discrimination and intuitive wisdom. It is therefore our discerning faculty of mind. It is the seat where we tap into our creativity and imagination, and where we make the most sensible decisions that are of benefit to one and all. Realistically, we cannot always be certain we are operating from our highest intellect. However, the opportunity to learn and become wiser from our errors is part of the maturation of the mind and the refinement of buddhi.

This higher mind can be tainted by the samskaras, which can project the past onto our present without our awareness. Again, samskaras are those deeply engrained mental imprints that formed from past experiences. They are projections that inhibit our clarity and create personality traits. They can also have a positive influence, however, leading us toward useful inclinations in life. Samskaras are generally considered to be the accumulated residues of our previous actions or dispositional tendencies, and they can lead toward the development of very specific desires, habits, and strong inclinations called vasanas. Vasanas are the latent psychological tendencies that, often unconsciously, drive us to seek out certain experiences in life, including particular relationships. However, the path of yoga aims to assist us in cultivating clear vision and *tarka*, or "discernment," through dissolving the samskaras and vasanas slowly over time.

Operating from the intelligence of the buddhi mind requires detached observation and emotional neutrality. The buddhi mind is aware of the impermanence of life and promotes emotional stability. It is a part of the vijnanamaya kosha. In its highest state, buddhi is reflected by self-observation without attachment, alignment with a cosmic intelligence, equanimous perception and disposition, and a cultivation of meditative awareness.

In addition to charting this anatomical map of the subtle mind, it is valuable to bring light to the concept of the *gunas*. In terms of the popular yogic belief around the creation of the universe (as we know it), the presence of the three gunas is a result of the equilibrium disturbance of prakriti. Prakriti, in this context, is the germinal state of material nature. Due to this disturbance, we now have the universe in a manifest state, with the three gunas in constant flux. They are creating and sustaining the cyclical nature of all that exists. The gunas govern all of the material world and therefore also the quality of the mind. They are specifically connected to the ahamkara. A translation of the Sanskrit word *guna* means "attribute." These *maha* gunas are *tamas*, *rajas*, and *sattva*.

Tamas is essential to life, despite often being considered something to transcend or diminish. Tamas relates to the earth element, the senses, the five elements, and therefore all that is dense and tangible in life. Tamas grounds and stabilizes. It is reflected in gravitational pull. However, especially as it pertains to the mind, tamas creates lethargy, inertia, dullness, and even depression. The major qualities of tamas are darkness, delusion, and death. It veils or obstructs higher consciousness. It brings about stagnation and decay.

Rajas aids us in moving out of tamas. It relates to activity, energy, passion, and variability. A rajasic mind is often goal oriented, driven, agitated, and tempted by sensory enjoyment. While these qualities of stimulation, movement, and motivation are required (to a degree) for all life to exist, rajas generally promotes a disintegration of the mind over time. It is intimately related to tamas, for when rajas is in excess the mind can fall into dullness instead of progressing to the higher state of *sattva*. If the mind is in a state of ongoing turbulence and excess activity, as when experiencing anxiety, for example, rajas often builds until the mind drops into immense exhaustion and dullness to numb out the intensity and avoid overwhelm. The rajasic mind is generally regarded as a more evolved state than tamas. However, it still keeps us bound to attachments and the qualities of ahamkara.

Sattva is the highest state of the three gunas. While it may appear to transcend rajas and tamas, we could see it as a perfect balance of the two, given they are both essential for life to function and exist. The Sanskrit word *sattva* translates to "true essence," "nature," "wisdom," "existence," "reality," and "good sense." Within the Samkhya philosophy specifically, it means "purity" or "goodness." Sattva creates harmony and balance. It is reflected in adaptability, clarity, contentment, luminosity, and peacefulness. Pure sattva is virtuous and devotional without any attachment or desire. A sattvic mind, cultivated by certain practices, diet, and lifestyle choices, is emotionally equanimous and anchored in love.

In the Yoga Sutras of Patanjali, we learn of two essential terms to unravel to aid us in mental self-mastery. These pertain directly to mastering *vrttis*, or mental modifications. Sutra 1.12, "*abhyasa vairagyabhyam tannirodhah*," reveals the indispensable concepts of *abhyasa* and *vairagya* as the imperative means to bringing any unsteadiness of the mind under control. *Abhyasa* refers to practice, but more specifically it implies a *consistent* practice of yoga. *Vairagya* indicates contemplative dispassion, nonattachment, and the absence of desire, where realistic. Therefore, it is the application of dedicated, consistent, uninterrupted practice (which moves us toward one-pointed concentration), alongside emotional neutrality and detachment from objects and outcomes, that leads us to discriminative wisdom. This is where we need to engage in tapas, a deeper level of self-discipline and perseverance. As a result, when any afflictions of the mind arise via our sensory experience of the world—that is, through manas and ahamkara, in addition to the influence of our samskaras—they quickly dissipate.

According to book two of the Yoga Sutras, entitled *Sadhana Pada*, there are five main afflictions of the mind that produce suffering and impede our progress. These are the kleshas, which include *avidya* (ignorance), *asmita* (egotism), *raga* (desire), *dvesha* (aversion), and *abhinivesha* (clinging to worldly life). By allowing ourselves to readily fall prey to these states of mind we only continue to develop deeper samskaras in addition to cultivating new karmas.

Avidya is often regarded as the root cause of the other four kleshas. Most commonly translated as "ignorance," it refers to our lack of awareness of the true nature of reality. As a result of a misperception of the external world and oneself, suffering arises.

Asmita, as previously noted, relates to the misidentification with the individual self. As a result, this perspective fuels a sense of separateness and disconnection from the Supreme Reality, or that which is fundamentally all-encompassing and ultimately formless.

Raga relates to desire and our preferences. More specifically, it reflects the attachment we have to pleasure, to the things we like. It is associated with both conscious and subconscious craving, which, when unmet, leaves us suffering. Think about how easy it is to waste hours of our life on screen time, trying to avoid the perceived pain of doing the things we know we should. Raga arises when we avoid supposed unpleasant experiences, many of which may be beneficial for us (or others), so we can indulge in what we like or whatever makes us feel good momentarily. It is also reflected in the constant need to please others.

Dvesha has a close bond with raga. It relates to aversion and the things we dislike, or even hate. In life, just as with pleasure, we can very easily be attached to pain and to the things that we do not like. This is due to our mental conditioning and bad habits. Consider how easy and commonplace it is to habitually eat the foods (or the amount of food) we know will leave us feeling unwell. Overcoming both raga and dvesha is a means to serving our future self, who will be thankful, and better off, in the long term.

Abhinivesha relates to a deeply embedded clinging to life, rooted in a fear of impermanence or death. This circles back to avidya and asmita. It is connected to our false sense of reality. Every human being knows they will inevitably die one day, yet it is a fear that we hold, mostly because of our delusion associated with the previous four kleshas. With its desire to be recognized and to have a sense of control at all times, our ego has a strong hold on us.

Patanjali offers us some guidance on how to overcome our mental afflictions, or kleshas. These include a consistent spiritual practice that cultivates tapasya (self-discipline), the study of yoga shastra (scripture) to gain knowledge of the Self (*svadhyaya*), and *Ishvarapranidhana* (surrendering to the Supreme). If our yoga practice—one that goes beyond the asana—is working, we begin to slowly overcome the kleshas. Our studentship draws back the veil of each affliction to reveal a more integrated awareness of both the uncertainty of each moment and all of existence, alongside the illumination of our eternal nature that transcends the body and mind.

As a final contemplation on the mind, I will add that not only are our thoughts both a reflection and *creator* of samskaras, but they also consequently drive our actions in the world. In turn, this creates new karma and new samskaras for each of us. Our individual circumstances are a reflection of accumulated karma, of both this and past lives. *Karma* translates from Sanskrit to "action." In this context, it indicates past actions that yield inevitable reactions and outcomes. However, it is the way we manage our karma—which most often relates to the way we mentally perceive and thereby respond to our circumstances—that ultimately dictates the outcome of everything we do (or don't do). Consider that immoral thoughts drive certain behavior, and that behavior is an action that causes a reaction.

In addition to the imprints already set in motion via existing samskaras, vasanas, and karmas, the mind significantly shapes our reality. These mental residues are what bridge the time between cause and effect. Yet the mind can also be utilized as a tool to resolve and transcend these impressions and conditions. As we come to understand, through the teachings of yoga, that karma as causal law is an ethical element to *samsara* (the process of rebirth), we can appreciate that all of these concepts around the mind are what ideally guide us to live a moral, studious, and virtuous life. People of most Indic traditions—Hindus, Buddhists, and Jains, for example—have long inquired into the way to minimize, if not eliminate, the source of karma and the resulting cycle of samsara. Yogananda points toward the truth of this human conundrum as a reminder that the deeper, subtle teachings of yoga hold the key to our freedom:

> Seeds of past karma cannot germinate if they are roasted in the fires of divine wisdom.[2]

The relationship between the physical and subtle anatomy is bidirectional. The bodies and layers of self directly influence each other at all times. In our current world, where we are so heavily attentive to Western anatomy and physiology in yoga (likely due to the emphasis on asana), it can feel challenging to understand, contemplate, and visualize how we can be in a tangible relationship with the subtle energy body. Intellectual knowledge will only take us so far. Although there are variations to the subtle anatomy across the numerous Indian traditions, generally we see that our understanding of this aspect of the self is populated with symbolism and metaphor. All of this can appear deeply mystical and even paradoxical at times.

The word *subtle* denotes something fine, delicate, and elusive. For those who have grown up in a world detached from these seemingly abstract ideas, it is fair to feel as if it is all quite nebulous. Given that the mention of the subtle body dating back to the Upanishads is somewhat cryptic, it is natural to feel we must decode the metaphysical on an intellectual level to a certain degree. If we are then able to stay anchored in a place of curiosity, wonder, and inquiry, we can begin to unravel the perceived complexities. As with anything in yoga, this requires direct practice. It requires a relationship to and engagement in the subtle. When we are truly working in this realm, all constructs of ideas and labels tend to fall away, and the abstract becomes palpable. Further into the book, we will explore these practical applications that take us inward through the various veneers of ourselves.

In yogic thought, the subtle anatomy is part of what animates us. Much of the more intricate esoteric anatomical features noted here are inextricably tied to Tantra, which, as we uncovered in chapter one, has profoundly impacted yoga as we know it today. Tantra very much solidified the subtle body theory as we know it. Classical yoga tends to place more emphasis on the koshas, prana, and the nadis. It is in both Tantra and Hatha yoga that we see all the other subtle anatomy discussed in greater depth.

Across the board, yoga traditions see the body as a temple, both literally and figuratively. It is our instrument for spiritual growth. When we delve into a yoga practice that illuminates the subtle terrain, we are essentially taking a pilgrimage throughout the body. In most Indic traditions, certain localities and sites of our microcosm are regarded as *tirthas*. A tirtha is a sacred pilgrimage location, both external and internal. It is often, although not always, a site near water. The human body is made up of approximately 60 percent water, so this is certainly fitting with respect to the internal veneration yoga invites us into. This focus on the subtle body is also of significance within Taoism, Buddhism, and Jainism.

Stereotypically, classical yoga takes a perspective toward the *physical* body that encourages detachment from sensory pleasure and a degree of aversion toward the body, potentially culminating in bodily transcendence. In contrast, Tantra invites us to embrace—and then eventually transmute—worldly enjoyment and our physical manifestation. Both offer value to the everyday householder. With their differences, they also overlap in many ways and have evident reverence toward the value of the subtle yogic anatomy. Yet some schools and systems see the subtle body as another obstacle to realization, and as a result they show little interest in pursuing it. Using this kind of reflection can aid us in pondering our own path and trajectory within yoga. Across the board, yoga exists to cast light on how we can both be in this world and simultaneously transcend it. It teaches us how to harness our vessel so we can, at the very least, have a glimmer of an experience into the fundamental essence of our individual highest Self. Whether we choose a path that aims to deploy or dismiss the physical and metaphysical anatomy, the final destination of yoga remains the same.

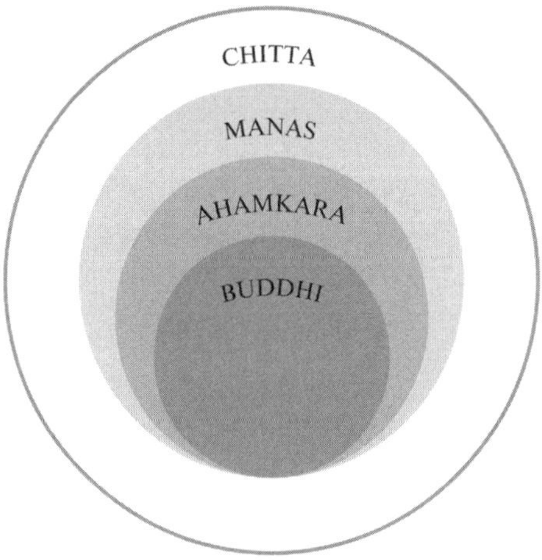

FIGURE 3. Major aspects of the mind

CONTEMPLATIONS

What aspects of my personal yoga practice, if any, regularly tend to the subtle anatomy?

What thoughts and behaviors do I engage in that are habitual and are possibly deeply engrained samskaras?

What mental and emotional responses of mine reflect the reactivity of manas or ahamkara?

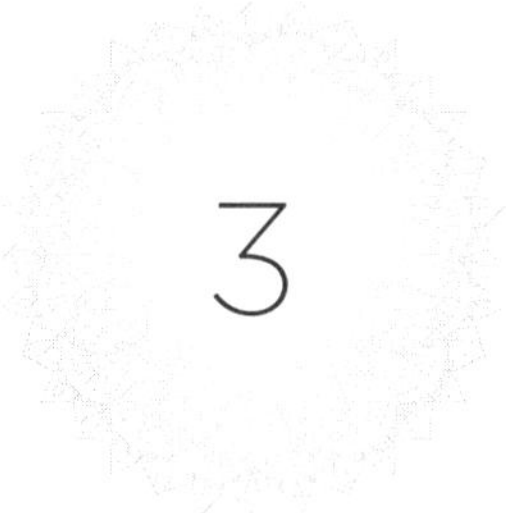

3

MARGA

WALKING THE PATH

TO EMBARK ON A PATH OF YOGA, and to allow the teachings to pervade all aspects of daily life, is no small undertaking. The mainstream perception of "advanced" yoga reflects intense and complex calisthenics, usually performed with excessive force—a path that is oriented solely outward. Unfortunately, too often this is a misguided grasp at external validation, as we see demonstrated across various social media platforms. In truth, what has traditionally been regarded as advanced and the most supreme path is a pursuit of the subtle, refined yogic knowledge that holds the potential to reveal the highest wisdom. However, it is only through persistent, attentive effort and reflective embodiment that we can even *begin* to climb a ladder to the highest states. Not many who are engaged in the current yoga trends are sincerely invested in leaning into the discomfort that can then be uprooted through an exploration of the deep inner terrain.

In 1929 the Indian philosopher, speaker, and mystic Jiddu Krishnamurti (1895–1986), stood in front of a large audience of thousands to share what came to be known as "Truth Is a Pathless Land" or the

"Dissolution Speech." A small passage from this talk holds wisdom and relevance that could inspire any seeker who is considering the pursuit of higher yoga:

> Truth cannot be brought down, rather the individual must make the effort to ascend to it. You cannot bring the mountain-top to the valley. If you would attain to the mountain-top you must pass through the valley, climb the steeps, unafraid of the dangerous precipices.

Not everyone is willing to ascend to the heights of yoga in this lifetime, but that is not to diminish the views from the valley; there is value at every stage. Any individual's karma will play a part in the teachers and the teachings they gain access to. A Vedic astrology chart is one of many traditional tools used to glean the direction of one's spiritual pursuits, karmas, and dharma. Another, lesser-known form of divination used to gaze into an individual's potential path is *samudrika shastra*, or the "knowledge of body features." This can include Vedic palmistry (*hasta samudrika*) and face-reading (*mukha samudrika*), for example. Simply put, samudrika shastra sees every physical mark or trait on a person to be an indicator of their divine destiny. Some *lakshanas* (characteristic features or qualities) are also believed to be highly auspicious.

Lineage and the Guru

What is lineage-based yoga? Ultimately, all yoga comes from someone, somewhere, at some point in time. Therefore, is not all yoga lineage based? Traditionally, a lineage denoted a connection to a living guru, one who passed on to the student certain teachings of a particular tradition—and only when the aspirant was deemed ready by the teacher. *Guru-shishya parampara* is the term to describe this unbroken chain of teachings; *parampara* is a Sanskrit word meaning "an uninterrupted series," "succession," "tradition," "lineage," or "continuation." The significant connotation here is *uninterrupted*. These days we can cherry-pick whatever aspect of yoga we wish to focus on—at least, any that has not been closely guarded by tradition. This guru-shishya (teacher-student) parampara not only refers to an unbroken thread of pure, undiluted, unadulterated teachings but also indicates a relationship that almost always included formal initiation of some kind. In which case, the teacher is regarded as the *díksha* (DEEK-shah, meaning "initiation") guru.

In this traditional setting, the student most commonly has little to no influence or say regarding what they learn or the teachings offered. Monetary payment is not usually requested by a spiritual guru, at least not in former times. However, the student may live with their teacher and serve them in other ways: cleaning their home, preparing meals, and perhaps even massaging the guru's feet (in the case of a dance guru, for example). The guru is remunerated, but more commonly through service or with gifts. This is *gurudakshina*. One may be automatically granted a guru through their own family. For example, this would be when someone's parents have a spiritual guru, and hence the children of the family acquire the same guru. Alternatively, a guru may be found purely by a chance occurrence or divine intervention. As the saying goes, "When the student is ready, the teacher will appear." Naturally, due to the globalization of yoga, this traditional and cultural approach to lineage-based teaching is not only less common but also realistically much more difficult to access.

The Sanskrit word *guru* is more commonly translated to suggest "darkness to light" (*gu* = darkness, *ru* = light). We can imagine that the teacher guides the student from the darkness of delusion to illumination. However, the word translates literally to "heavy." So perhaps the more appropriate interpretation of *guru* would be to imagine that the student—who lacks a *consistent* relationship to the earth element and therefore lacks stability—is anchored by the teacher, who then connects them with reality. The Supreme Reality, that is. Heavy with knowledge, the guru is a conduit to the Supreme. The guru brings the disciple into greater steadiness and clarity. But the student must be stable of mind first. This type of guru can be called the *satguru*—a personal guru who assists in aligning the student with the ultimate truth of reality. We could say that they act like a benefactor. This relationship is where the teacher induces *shravana*. Through deep, attentive listening by the student, shravana is the hearing of sacred secrets from the yogic teachings that are being revealed directly from the guru. This includes being able to hear the correct recitation of Sanskrit pronunciation, which imparts its own potent mystical benefits.

Ideally, a guru is a vessel for the timeless and infallible teachings to come through. However, in human form any guru will have their limitations. No doubt many have fallen from grace—both those of India and of the Western world. As a result, a vast number of spiritual practitioners have entirely thrown away any belief in the value of the guru. Sadly, too many have been deceived or deluded by fraudulent and often promiscuous gurus. Then, having lost their sense of sovereignty and discernment, disciples and devotees who have experienced oppression and peer pressure are left no apparent choice but to stay silent. This has tarnished and discredited the invaluable gift of transformative guidance that can be received from a potential guru.

The guru-shishya relationship should not be a codependent one. A student's autonomy and clear discrimination must be intact. This is because, fundamentally, the commitment to one's guru requires wholehearted faith. The Sanskrit term *shraddha* denotes trust, faith, and reverence. It reflects a state of humility and unwavering respect toward the guru. Embodied as a deeply internal attitude, it develops with time and ongoing inquiry. As a student attentively listens, applies, and witnesses yogic teachings unfolding, divine truths are revealed, and our trust or belief is further solidified. Our dedication and commitment become unshakable. This is not some kind of blind faith or ignorance. Lineage and the guru can hold us as we traverse the inner terrain and subsequent transformations. Parampara aids us in the necessary steps required to mature along the path. It can offer a more efficient and easeful journey of evolution, one that further moves us toward the potential of experiencing *sharanagati* (sha-ra-NAH-gati), a total surrender that is free from any sense of clinging.

One of the most well-known guru mantras, and one that speaks to the broader aspect of guru, not just as a direct teacher in human form, is the opening of the Guru Stotram from the *Guru Gita*:

> GURURBRAHMA GURURVISHNUH GURURDEVO MAHESHVARAH |
> GURUSSAKSHAT PARAMBRAHMA TASMAI SHRIGURAVE NAMAH ||
>
> The guru is Brahma, Visnu and Siva. The guru is unquestionably the supreme Brahman (essence of all), to that guru, my salutations.[3]

Guru Purnima is an auspicious annual occasion to honor and celebrate one's guru and teachers. The Sanskrit word *purnima* refers to the full moon. The date normally falls on a full moon in the month of July. More specifically, it is the full moon in the lunar constellation of

Ashadha Nakshatra in Vedic astrology. Across various yoga traditions, seekers often honor the legendary sage Veda Vyasa during this occasion. It is also believed to be the anniversary of when Lord Shiva—the *adiyogi*—shared the knowledge of yoga to the *Saptarishi* (seven sages), who went on to disseminate this wisdom to the world. On Guru Purnima we pay respect to all of our teachers. In the Indian culture, this traditionally includes our parents also, especially our mother.

The Lord of Yoga

As one of the three gods in the venerated *Trimurti* (tree-MOOR-tee), Shiva is revered as the undeniable *adiyogi* (AH-dee-yogi), the first yogi. Worshipped as an omniscient being, he lives an ascetic life. Shiva is also a householder, married with children—one of whom is the idolized Ganapati, or Ganesha. His cosmic vehicle, or *vahana*, is Nandi the bull, who represents ultimate strength. Mount Kailash (located in Tibet) is his summer abode. Kashi (otherwise known as Benares or Varanasi) is his winter dwelling place. Shiva embodies a compassionate and patient quality—steady, eternal, pure, and unruffled. As this *original* yogi, he represents a state of the eternal silent witness. It is held that Shiva, said to be the teacher of all teachers, the guru of all gurus, was the first to share the knowledge and teachings of yoga. The first student to receive his wisdom was, of course, his consort, Parvati. Parvati is said to be a reincarnation of Shiva's first wife, Sati, who immolated herself in a holy sacrificial fire after her father's disapproval of their marriage.

Shiva, like all Sanskrit words, has a number of meanings and uses. Some common translations of the word are "auspicious," "benevolent," "favorable," "liberation," "time," and "emancipation." These allude to the overarching nature and qualities of Lord Shiva. He manifests in various personified forms that each express a varied spectrum of attributes and character. For example, Rudra is his fierce form, representing the destruction and decay that is required for new life and creation to emerge. Rudra is the violent and wild storm-god who expresses violence specifically for purposes of the highest good. Kala Bhairava is an even more fearsome form of Shiva.

Nataraja may be the most well-known form of Shiva, revered in the classical performing arts of India. This Lord (Raja) of Dance is depicted in movement (called *tandava*) within a ring of fire, treading on a dwarf (who represents the ego), with wildly arranged, matted hair, holding a *damaru* drum in his upper right hand (representing cosmic sound or the rhythm of the beating heart). His presence teaches us of the cycle of creation and destruction, or birth and death. One of the most revered Shiva mantras that has been commonly recited for centuries is the *Mahamrtyunjaya*:

> OM TRYAMBAKAM YAJAMAHE SUGANDHIM PUSHTIVARDHANAM |
> URVARUKAMIVA BANDHANAN MRTYOMUKSHIYA MA'MRTAAT ||
>
> *We worship the three-eyed One, who is fragrant and the increaser of nourishment. May we be freed from bondage and death—just as the ripened melon falls from the vine—and that we be granted the nectar of immortality.*[4]

The iconographical portrayal of Lord Shiva most suitable to the path of yoga is that of the *mahayogi* (great yogi) Yogeshvara. Here he is seated in his benevolent and patient state. His attention waning, or moving inward, is symbolically indicated by the crescent moon on his forehead. His third eye, representing knowledge, is closed. When open, it destroys every facet of material existence, as all Shiva sees is nonduality. His hair is matted, looking like dreadlocks or cowry shells, as a display of non-attachment. Ganga, as the cosmic waters, was brought down to earth via Shiva's head to reduce her turbulent force. As a result, all the energy of the galaxy is falling down on his head. Ganga was tamed within his matted locks, eventually landing down in the Himalayas, where still today she is continually led through Haridwar, Varanasi, and eventually to the ocean. Shiva's body smeared all over with ashes—representing death—alludes to what was incinerated and has thereby been stabilized. His throat, where he holds poison and transmutes it, is blue in color, demonstrating self-mastery.

Shiva, as the mahayogi, also holds the damaru drum as a symbol of our mortality, the beating heart or rhythm of life, alongside the sound creation of Sanṣkrit. Shiva's *trishula*, or trident, reflects the sacred trinities, such as the three gunas, doshas, major nadis, and so forth. He wears a necklace made of holy *rudraksha* seeds and a tiger skin. He is adorned with serpents around his waist that represent his power. The naga Vasuki (king of the nagas, serpent-like semidivine beings) is around his neck, symbolizing Shiva's immense self-control. A dhyana *shloka* found in the *Abhinaya Darpanam*, a Sanskrit treatise on classical Indian dance, alludes to Shiva's physical features and form:

> ANGIKAM BHUVANAM YASYA |
> VACIKAM SARVA VANMAYAM ||
> AHARYAM CHANDRATARADI |
> TVAM NAMAH SATTVIKAM SHIVAM ||
>
> *The movement of whose body is the world, whose speech the sum of all language,*
> *Whose jewels are the moon and stars—to that pure Shiva I bow!*[5]

The gods that constitute the Trimurti correspond to the three gunas of tamas (Shiva), rajas (Brahma), and sattva (Vishnu). With his affiliation to tamas, Shiva is associated with alcohol and all intoxicating drugs. He helps us find a way to overcome and transcend the things that dull and darken our mind and spirit. Tamas also correlates to heaviness, stability, and groundedness. Gravity is a fine example of the essential nature of tamas in the material realm. This ties back to the translation of *guru* as that which grounds and steadies us. Remember, Shiva is the ultimate guru of gurus, after all.

Addressing the "Lord of Yoga" would not be complete without acknowledging the immense influence of another Yogeshvara, Lord Krishna. In the Vaishnava—or Bhakti yoga—tradition in particular, Krishna is held in highest esteem. This is primarily through his teachings found within the Mahabharata and the *Bhagavata Purana* (also known as the *Shrimad Bhagavatam*). He is one of the ten avatars of the supreme deity, Vishnu. Krishna's teachings on yoga are deeply relatable to the average yoga practitioner. Through story, we witness the most supreme teachings woven through the chaos of householder life. These stories convey the wisdom applicable to how we live each day and to our relationship with the divine. Krishna assists us in assimilating and alchemizing the complexities of worldly life. He moves us into spiritual growth through action, i.e., karma and dharma. Like Shiva's, blue is often the color of his skin,

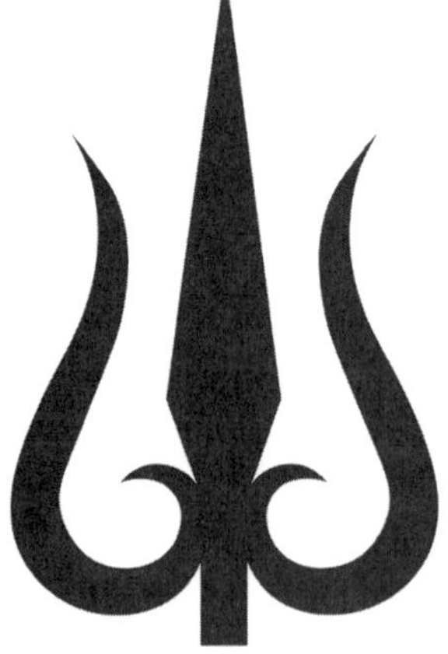

FIGURE 4. A trident which is attributed to Lord Shiva (and the Goddess Durga). It is also a symbol that represents the Trimurti, along with other auspicious trinities such as the three gunas, the three doshas, etc.

which symbolizes his expansive nature—just like the vast blue sky or the ocean. He is often seen with a peacock feather, which indicates beauty and knowledge (the peacock is also present-day India's national bird).

All of the iconographical representations of deities within the Indic teachings exist to help us realize eternal truths, ethics, and what is beyond the mundane. Their symbols and stories have the capacity to guide us and provide refuge from the turbulence of human existence. While they are often revered and worshipped as religious figures, their teachings transcend doctrine. After all, "Hinduism" is an umbrella term rather than a word that denotes a specific path or belief system. The term *Hindu* encompasses Shakta, Shaiva, and Vaishnava traditions, along with many others. Presentation of the Supreme can be expressed in various ways, though imparting the same fundamental message. In this sense, spirituality and eternal truths transcend religious ideas and application.

Tradition

Let's begin by stating what is likely evident at this point. There is no one single tradition of yoga exclusively. Just like India as a nation, yoga is a "melting pot." To explore the historical timeline of yoga, as chapter one aims to do, we no doubt affirm this further. When there are a multitude of paths, practices, and persons to learn from, it can be a challenge to determine what is anchored in authenticity. What it is that makes something traditional in yoga can no doubt be argued. However, a relatively objective perspective would regard traditional yoga as rooted in longstanding customs, cultural heritage, and the oral history of parampara. Therefore, we could say that tradition is tied to lineage. Even still, throughout the extensive history of yoga, many teachers and gurus at times must have adapted certain principles or techniques after assimilating them.

It is a popular claim these days that certain techniques or practices are "lineage based" and thereby anchored in tradition. Often it seems like a selling point, and it can be misleading marketing. How can we genuinely claim that our path or practice is lineage based? Ultimately, all yoga-related teachings come from someone, somewhere, at some point in time. Even if those teachings are innovated upon and seem "new," they are ultimately founded on something that is not new. Therefore, no one could claim to own yoga; it is something beyond ownership. However, it must be reiterated that yoga originates from, and is indigenous to, the Indian subcontinent (and its amalgamation of cultures).

Clarity and insight into tradition—through the lens of yoga specifically—may be revealed through the essence of *sampradaya* (sum-pra-DAH-ya). *Sampradaya* is the Sanskrit word used to imply tradition. It speaks to the transmission of teachings from guru to seeker. *Sampradaya* refers to a *living* tradition or lineage. This suggests that there is a very clear succession of generations. This is not a kind of "pick and choose" approach to learning, where we make our own (yogic) salad to suit our personal taste. It is an approach that holds steady an undiluted and unbroken thread of continuity with the past.

Sampradaya presents an authority and stewardship that is upheld and respected. It does not fall prey to trends, and it does not need to be sold or marketed in the public eye. It gives us specific tools and techniques that are individualized to our needs, rather than feeding our desire to take what we want and then leave. It asks a long-term commitment, steeped in patience and reverence. Dedication to a sampradaya should be mutually beneficial and not transactional. The living lineage and guru act as a kind of midwife, supporting each adherent to enliven the robust wisdom teachings within. In return, the loyal student ensures that the insights are not only retained, but resiliently flourish over the long-term.

Understandably, a large percentage of sincere seekers on the path of yoga may never come to be immersed and initiated in sampradaya, especially those outside of the Indian subcontinent. This should not limit anyone's capacity to be a recipient and steward of the teachings, however. As pilgrims on the path, we must seek out the teachers and teachings that inspire *smarana*—a "remembrance" or "calling to mind" of our sacred highest Self. To see the path as a lifelong *yatra* (YAH-trah, meaning "pilgrimage"), we can trust it will be sprinkled with auspicious moments and junctures. Humbly and patiently, the sadhaka awaits the revelations that come only through dedicated study and practice.

Four Aims of Life

From the most revered text of Ayurveda, the following quote (or sutra) notes that the fundamental aims of life—*dharma*, *artha*, *kama*, and *moksha*—are attained only through good health:

> DHARMARTHAKAMAMOKSHANAMAROGYAṂ MULAM UTTAMAM || [6]

This could be loosely translated to suggest that optimal health is the *foundation* required to cultivate and pursue duty, prosperity, pleasure, and ultimate freedom. It is an absence of disease that is the substratum that enables us to pursue these four *purushartha*. Through this understanding we can further appreciate how yoga and Ayurveda are inherently intertwined. Usually described as aims or goals for life, on the surface the purusharthas are general objectives for humankind. Taught or alluded to within several venerated texts, such as the Mahabharata and the *Ramayana*, each of these four themes can give us, as householders, a useful framework for how we could ideally orchestrate our lives. Especially when applied with an awareness of the manner and order in which they are more commonly presented, the purusharthas provide useful guidance to help us anchor into the cultural heritage of yogic teachings.

For those who choose to *not* renounce worldly life, allowing the four aims of dharma, artha, kama, and moksha to direct their path can be of immense solace. In the vast sea of systems, sects, techniques, and teachings, confusion is generally overcome for any seeker who has cultivated steady direction and boundaries for their spiritual and worldly life to flourish within. Author, Ayurvedic physician, and mentor to many in the fields of Tantra, Jyotisha, and beyond, Dr. Robert Svoboda speaks to this present-day relevance of the four guiding aims:

> If you're following your path through life properly; if you have aligned yourself with the material world in the right way, in order to follow that path properly; if you're fulfilling the desires that are legitimate and that you strongly hold and want to fulfill, then the likelihood is you will not be too much deluded.[7]

DHARMA

Your innate purpose and path, whereby you feel a longing and devotion toward your life's work, is likened to dharma. Ultimately, dharma is what uplifts society in some way—both the people and the planet. It is about upholding and sustaining the natural cosmic order through all that we do. Through the pursuit of dharma, we can tap into uncapped inherent creativity and contentment. Dharma is any kind of work for the sake of posterity and service (which is not always the same as charity). If you were some kind of quiet superhero undercover, contemplate what may be your greatest assignment in life and how you could best facilitate that. Consider that dharma does not need to come with accolades, awards, or rewards. Dharma does not require grasping or excessive striving. Dharma is often what calls to you, time and time again, even when life is challenging or you are distracted. Think of dharma as a verb, rather than a noun, a title, or a job. Dharma alludes to living in alignment with higher cosmic configurations.

While dharma is related to purpose, however, it is not always directly connected to what you may feel exclusively *passionate* about. This is an essential discernment. For example, someone may feel passionate about yoga and sharing yoga, but their dharmic purpose may not be to formally *teach* yoga. Things that we are passionate about may overlap with our dharma, but they may also relate more to kama—desires and things that bring pleasure. In addition, your individual dharma—*svadharma*—is not necessarily your *occupation*. The English language can often be limited in conveying the depth of Sanskrit terms, and even the word "purpose" may encourage excessive desire for achievement that takes us further away from aligning with our dharma. Miscomprehension of dharma can come with significant consequences for oneself and others. Dharma is not goal oriented. It represents who we fundamentally are and what we are here to do in this particular lifetime (which no doubt has a direct relationship to our karma and astrological arrangements).

Some pertinent questions to ask may be:

What is my most significant duty in life?

What is the one thing that feels profoundly meaningful?

Where is my most heartfelt sense of devotion directed?

What am I inherently good at?

Perhaps you have more than one dharmic duty at any given time, such as being a parent while simultaneously pursuing a significant community offering. Consider that your dharma, your duty, could be expressed through your current occupation, even if it is seemingly unrelated. While not deemed the easy path by any means, dharma does give us energy and generate resources. This leads us to the next purushartha.

ARTHA

Generally regarded as a by-product of pursuing dharma, artha emphasizes the value of cultivating a bountiful life through wealth of all kinds. Artha is not only the generation of monetary wealth or value. It is also the acquisition of abundant resources that assist us in pursuing a balanced and healthy life so we can continue to pursue our dharma for the good of all. In a sense, dharma and artha are inseparable and fuel each other. Accruing an appropriate degree of wealth or resources is what ensures we can take care of ourselves and others. It aids us in being able to provide for our loved ones and, if we have children, to raise and teach another generation. Aside from financial gains, artha traditionally referred to obtaining land, food, and having children (to ensure one would be cared for later in life).

Artha in our present-day world usually relates to sustenance, health, and financial security. Without these in place, we all experience immense stress and cannot pursue our worldly duties. Even with spiritual and charitable work, we must ensure our basic needs are met. Without having established security and stability, we cannot move through life and engage in any aspirations or activity, such as our education, an occupation, relationships, or general pleasures and fruitful worldly enjoyment. An abundance of health and resources enables us to contribute greatly to our immediate and wider community. The absence of disease and our financial security impact the nervous system, which gives us the strength, resilience, and inspiration to create and serve. If we experience ill health or financial struggle, we cannot direct energy or attention beyond the sympathetic state of survival.

In the Vedic householder tradition, being established in the cultivation of artha is expected. At the same time, we are discouraged from greed and excess. Therefore, a higher level of wealth, security, and resources is ideally carefully and spiritually directed. Money and resources are forms of shakti, so how we choose to employ, circulate, and steward these in society impacts our individual and collective karma. More wealth brings more responsibility. An appreciation for the things we already have can anchor us into the essence of artha and break the societal conditioning of materialism. Living a simple life—where basic needs are met, health is intact, and we are also graciously remunerated appropriately for our worth in our work—does not have to be devoid of pleasure. This kind of life can be a profoundly wholesome and spiritual one.

KAMA

With integrity and virtue, we can and should enjoy the pleasures of life. Kama—not *karma*—means "pleasure" and "enjoyment." This is not an advocation of indulgence or attachment. When we are taking care of our duties and responsibilities, we can then direct attention toward the things we also like to do and enjoy. It is here that we recognize the immense blessing of being born into human form. It is only through our *human* existence that we can pursue a spiritual path, whether we chose to renounce worldly desires very early on or not. If immersed in the householder tradition, we are to embrace and enjoy the present moment and all that comes with it. This includes appreciating sights, sounds, smells, tastes, and experiences—without craving. Feeling our connection with nature, appreciating every sunrise and the blossoming of a flower, or pausing to witness the most miraculous and seemingly simple things—this is kama. Kama invites us to enjoy the fruits of our efforts. Society today is so fast-paced that we rarely stop to appreciate or celebrate the joys and successes. Through the teachings of kama, we are encouraged to pause and experience the beauty around us. Overindulgence, selfishness, egocentricity, obsession, addiction, and attachment are not kama. Kama, when embraced genuinely with modesty, promotes presence and reverence.

MOKSHA

The first three purusharthas lay a foundation for this last aim, moksha. It is one that we generally come to later in life, once we have a sense of completing our worldly commitments. When we experience a contentment toward worldly duties that promotes closure, the only thing left to do is to go within. At this point, there is a distinct sense of fulfillment and, as a result, an inclination to retract from society. Typically, moksha is said to be "liberation." While this is the highest attainment, given that moksha implies "freedom," we could say that it is also a slow releasing away from our actions in the world. Throughout our day-to-day, moksha is the creation or allowance of more space whereby, eventually, we hand over responsibilities and the need to generate more resources. It is a steady withdrawal. We could say that it is the culmination of the yogic pursuits and practices over the course of a lifetime. Moksha is freedom from craving of all kinds—recognition, labels, roles, pleasures, and aspirations. For some, one day it may be the liberation from identification with the individual self, even for a moment in time, that is, Self-realization.

Paths of Yoga

Bharata, or the ancient Indian subcontinent, houses a tremendous amount of diversity. Potentially immeasurable, the diversity within each area—languages, foods, textiles, traditions, philosophical and religious beliefs, customs, and arts—is astounding. Within India itself, a seemingly innumerable number of threads are woven together to make the tapestry that is the cultural hub of yoga today. As reflected in India's daily life, yoga as a path brimming with potential practices can be taken in many different directions. In most cases, these all eventually lead to the same destination. The Sanskrit word *marga* is often used to indicate the spiritual "path," "passage," "road," "way," or "journey" that a seeker is on. Exceedingly different from practicing modern-day styles of postural yoga, traditionally an aspirant would align with one certain system or path composed of identifiable principles, practices, and philosophical teachings. This was, and still is, a reflection of yoga embedded into every aspect of life, rather than being an isolated or compartmentalized practice.

Even the multiple paths of yoga that have stood the test of time reflect commonalities and overlaps, despite their notable differences. A very simple example of this is the core teachings of the Bhagavad Gita that present Bhakti, Karma, Jnana, and Raja yoga all threaded together. This section of the book aims to highlight the most common or accessible yogic paths. While their distinctions will be apparent, it is essential to emphasize that they do not contradict each other, generally speaking. They are interrelated. The path undertaken is usually related to the dharma, karma, and Jyotisha of the unique individual, if not prompted directly by a guru. In the end, we are all moving at our own pace toward the higher knowledge and ultimate destination of liberation.

BHAKTI YOGA

At the heart of the Bhakti path, one sees oneself as a devotee of the Supreme in the form of a particular deity—often Krishna, but certainly not always. Puja and all forms of worship are an essential aspect of daily life and are performed with great sincerity. For example, it is believed that all forms of Vishnu love *alamkara* (which is to decorate and adorn the *murti*, or idol), and all forms of Shiva love *abhisheka* (which is to bathe and anoint the murti). Food is offered to the deity and is later distributed and consumed as *prasad* (something that has been consecrated). Singing and listening to *bhajans* and participation in *kirtanam*—repetition and glorification of names of the divine through storytelling and song—are commonplace acts of this devotional path.

Bhakti has a distinctly foundational attitude. A path open to all, with no eligibility criteria or set rules, it is a heart-centered life for those who either do not have access to or have less desire for traditional Veda study or elaborate rituals. Sanskrit mantra recitation is a big component of the Bhakti path. There are nine traditional methods of devotion that are implored, called *navadhabhakti*, such as salutations (*yandanam*), service to the divine (*dasyam*), friendliness (*sakhyam*), seeking shelter in the divine specifically through surrender (*atma nivedanam*), deep listening (*shravana*), contemplation (*smarana*), and puja or worship (*archana*). Often, on the Bhakti path one becomes intoxicated with joy, adoration, and a fundamental sense of satisfaction. The performance of all mundane worldly duties is offered to the divine. Personal desires are mostly surrendered and released. For the *bhakta*, every day is filled with unceasing inner prayer, as though there is uninterrupted contemplation on the divine.

Said to be best for Kali Yuga (the present age), Bhakti yoga is expressed outwardly in devotion, adoration, emotional love, and unwavering faith (shraddha) toward the Supreme. Inwardly, it is an unceasing awareness of our eternal true nature. The devotee is always inclined to ask, *In what way can I please the Supreme?* The bhakta can become derailed on the path if their devotion has not matured enough and thus excessive emotionalism arises in their relationship with others.

Around the world, the Hare Krishna movement is one of the largest established Bhakti yoga communities. Practitioners value deep and regular study of the *Srimad Bhagavatam* text, participation in *kirtan*, service to the deity (generally Lord Krishna or Lord Jagannatha) and their community, and recitation of the Hare Krishna mantra. Historically speaking, one of the most famous Bhakti saints was Purandara Dasa.

KARMA YOGA

Otherwise known as the "yoga of action," Karma yoga, or *Karma marga*, is a path of service and selfless acts that benefit others. This approach of doing our duty without egoic attachment is said to purify the mind. *Seva* is the central theme or teaching within Karma yoga, in which the seeker relinquishes immediate personal gratification or reward and extends their efforts outward for the good of their community or the planet. This path is anchored in ethics, non-attachment, and benevolence. It promotes a distinct neutrality toward loss and gain. Karma yoga involves dedicating time, effort, and finances to supporting other people and initiatives. It inspires a humbleness and mindfulness, and joy is experienced from rendering service to others. This kind of work is worship, for one on the Karma yoga path.

What Karma yoga does *not* ask of us, however, is to renounce our emotions or basic needs. Through Karma yoga, we are inspired to give from our contentment and overflow, not from a presumptuous desire to accrue good karma. Those drawn to the path inherently love to offer their time and energy to a greater mission. Natural renouncers, they find it easy to be generous with resources, and they experience immense joy from giving. Volunteering in the community causes great enthusiasm for anyone drawn to this path. Where possible, they embrace not only seva (which mostly encompasses offering time and energy) but also *dana*, which usually refers to the act of donating money, gifts, or resources.

Selfless service to the right cause is a form of worship and spiritual practice and is therefore steeped in reciprocity at the highest level only. This level of service should satiate the desire to be served in return. Therefore, an aspirant does not seek favors, rewards, or recognition. Failure to recognize others or taking credit for the positive fruits of one's actions can be a reflection of derailment from the essence of Karma yoga. Teachings on Karma yoga can be found in multiple texts, such as the Bhagavad Gita and the Bhagavad Purana.

JNANA YOGA

Often thought to be the accumulation of higher knowledge and wisdom, Jnana yoga is about deep inquiry into one's eternal nature and that which is beyond the mind. This path promotes the acquisition of revelations that draw us away from suffering and closer to liberation. It is a contemplative marga, engaging the intellect through refined discernment to uncover the truth of reality. Often misunderstood as an accrual of knowledge for the mere purpose of debate, Jnana yoga is intended to take our awareness inward and to prompt meditation on the question, *Who am I?*

On the surface level, this path requires a vast capacity for the development of *smriti*, or memory, due to a need for in-depth study, reflection, and contemplation. Suggested to be a slower path to realization when the focus is on the intellectual, Jnana marga asks us to ruminate in quietude. Founded on nondual philosophy, this path of higher knowledge begins with seemingly relentless study, inquiry, and discussion. Eventually the seeker is encouraged to create or allow distance from the mundane mind and to temper the influence of the sense organs. The drawback of Jnana yoga can be too much intellectualism, resulting in restlessness, arrogance, and skepticism. Any of these pitfalls can be a cause of derailment, hence the slower rate toward Self-realization.

KRIYA YOGA

The term "kriya yoga" is used across different contexts. For example, kriya yoga is mentioned within Patanjali's Yoga Sutras. It also relates to the use of purification kriyas in Hatha or kundalini yoga. Here, as it pertains to a path, Kriya yoga refers to any lineage that is directly traced back to the teachings of Lahiri Mahasaya (Shyama Charan Lahiri), disciple of the Himalayan yogi Mahavatara Babaji (Tryambaknath). Made most famous across the world by Paramahansa Yogananda via his book *Autobiography of a Yogi*, the transformative Kriya yoga techniques are closely guarded and require in-person initiation. There are many techniques called "kriya." The word itself means "action" and has the same root as *karma*. Therefore, it is important to emphasize that not all Kriya yoga relates to this particular school or lineage.

Employed by yogins, mystics, and rishis, the kriya practices have also been adapted to be accessible for the householder. The Kriya yoga system that is traced back to Lahiri Mahasaya utilizes various postures, pranayama, and meditation practices alongside a steady commitment to certain philosophical studies and a sattvic, vegetarian lifestyle. In the book *Kriya Yoga*, Paramahamsa Hariharananda states that "Kriya Yoga greatly reduces the time required for emancipation and makes it possible in one birth." Specific techniques are intended to direct and control the movement of prana in the body, as well as the cultivation of higher states of consciousness. Hariharananda goes on to share that "there are six stages of Kriya technique through which a *kriyavan* can control the different centers and get Self-realization."[8]

Practically speaking, in Kriya yoga emphasis is often placed on the use of Sanskrit mantra rumination and meditation, alongside working with the subtle spinal column through pranayama, sound, and contemplation. Through ritual and deliberate practices, the Kriya path also holds the sun and fire in highest esteem. Kriya yoga hones the subtle movement of prana in congruence with the breath with the aspiration to experience the mystical internal—and eternal—sound and light within.

MANTRA YOGA

On the initial level, this path is an undertaking of mantra sadhana—an internal recitation and rumination on a bija or Vedic mantra—thereby engaging in the awareness of *nada*, or cosmic sound. Here there is an imperative integration of the mind with prana. However, this path is not about mere intellectual understanding and repetition of Sanskrit mantras (although it may begin that way). With an appreciation that sound is the most subtle element of manifestation, from which everything has come forth, Mantra yoga requires that we uncover the deeper meaning of any mantra and then learn to place it specifically (nyasa) within the subtle body. Requiring initiation, this path uses mantra that is internally contemplated and used to purify or activate the energetic body. This ultimately leads to a cultivation of prana that is directed into a single point. It is within this technique that correct Sanskrit articulation is crucial. Tantrik in nature, Mantra yoga at its highest state has a direct relationship to that of *laya* yoga, the dissolution of the mind and ego identification.

HATHA YOGA

Contrary to what is usually promoted and offered in mainstream yoga studios across the globe, Hatha yoga is not a "style" of postural yoga. It is a system or path that utilizes various techniques and considerations that can be successfully woven into the context of a performative or physical yoga practice, but only when understood correctly and sincerely embodied. In the most simplistic sense, the Hatha yoga path has been influenced mostly by asceticism and Tantra. Importantly, it has heavily informed the yoga we know today. The word *hatha* means "force," and rightly so. Traditionally, Hatha has always been an austere path to undertake, with demanding techniques and great abstinences that may result in attainment of certain *siddhi* (magical powers). These powers, though, are not the fundamental goal. One of the most physical approaches to a yogic path, Hatha yoga incorporates the engagement of kriya, bandha, mudra, the largest selection of asanas (predating modern yoga styles), pranayama, pratyahara, the *shadchakra* (six major chakras), kundalini arousal, dharana, dhyana, and samadhi. This is all based on the assumption that the yamas and niyamas have already been tended to.

The goal within Hatha yoga is generally regarded to be reabsorption or dissolution of the mind (laya yoga) into the unmanifest state. This very subtle process utilizes nada (sound) as Sanskrit syllables, called bija, that are harnessed and placed (via the technique of nyasa) within the subtle body via a piercing of the chakras. This process ties back in to mantra yoga. Eventually, the sound merges into the eternal silence.

Hatha is more often simplistically translated as referring to sun (*ha*) and moon (*tha*). This speaks directly to the attention it places on the *pancha vayu.* Within this, Hatha yoga more specifically puts emphasis on the reversal and union of apana and prana vayu in the central channel of sushumna nadi. This is with a specific goal of cultivating the internal subtle fire and arousal of kundalini. It is these earlier, tangible techniques on the Hatha yoga path that are used to clear any bodily obstructions and cultivate effective circulation of prana. Eventually the path orients inward to develop more subtle sensitivities, ideally culminating in attainment of the higher state of Raja yoga where duality is dissolved. Some may say that Hatha yoga is the means and Raja yoga is the aim.

RAJA YOGA

Usually claimed be the most supreme of all paths, Raja yoga is taught as a system with various techniques and also as a state of being. *Raja yoga* can be used as a synonym for Patanjali's Ashtanga yoga, as laid out in his Yoga Sutras. Also called "classical yoga," this eight-limbed approach places far less importance on physical techniques—sometimes seemingly diminishing them—and instead focuses on the inwardly oriented meditative approach. Not to be confused with the ashtanga yoga of Pattabhi Jois, this well-known approach begins with the observances of yama and niyama, moving to asana (primarily as seated postures), pranayama, pratyahara, dharana, dhyana, and finally the (multileveled) state of samadhi. Swami Vivekananda is regarded as the main proponent of the connection between Patanjali's Ashtanga yoga—one of the six *darshanas*, or schools of philosophy—and Raja yoga.

The Sanskrit word *raja* (RAH-ja) translates to "king," "chief," "sovereign," or "best of its kind." Therefore, we can understand that Raja yoga is often upheld as the ultimate of all systems of yoga. Simultaneously, and depending on the context, *raja yoga* refers to a state of being—that is, the most supreme state where the individual self merges or reintegrates with the universal Self. It is deemed the ultimate goal, the most sovereign. This earlier understanding is reflected, for example, in Hatha yoga's proclamation that its systematic approach is the stairway to the attainment of raja yoga (as a state of being). "Raja yoga" in reference to a path, as in the case of the aforementioned "Ashtanga yoga," is generally believed to be retronym.

Modern Styles

With the proliferation of modern postural yoga—or transnational yoga—numerous distinct approaches to the physical techniques have arisen, some of which can be quite clearly traced back to earlier traditions of influence. Others carry a little more ambivalence. Regardless, it is undeniable that the modern body benefits from this often-performative application of yoga postures. For the most part, yoga "asanas" have developed out of a blend of martial forms, gymnastics, and other fitness trends. Even today there are some parallels with the classical dance and martial arts of India. These poses and movements serve to move prana more effectively, improve breathing capacity, quiet the mind, cultivate bodily awareness, and create a physical vessel that is able to sit in stillness for extended periods in meditation. Postural yoga should not be diminished. The health and comfortability of the physical body is paramount to introspective states. Simultaneously, we must remember that in isolation the poses themselves are not yoga. Especially when they are devoid of the more subtle, yet still physical, techniques such as bandha and mudra. Postural styles are one facet of yoga (although some traditionalists would understandably argue that even this is too generous). Either way, it is still beneficial to grasp an understanding of the various approaches or "styles" of postural yoga that have multiplied over the past century or two, especially given that postural yoga is the doorway to the path for most.

This section serves to purely offer a general overview of the most popularized styles of yoga. Keep in mind, it is not an exhaustive list nor is it presented in any hierarchical order. Also, at times the lines are blurred between a style of postural yoga and a particular tradition. Certain present-day *schools* of yoga, for example, have established a defining approach to techniques and practices that are undoubtedly founded on and developed from a longstanding tradition—usually Hatha yoga. In this case significant emphasis is placed on other yogic teachings beyond the physical poses (in addition to the postural applications). Some may argue that any one of the following styles are in fact multifaceted and inclusive of deeper aspects of yoga. While that may be true to a degree, the styles listed here are selected because they have become renowned specifically for their signature physical approach.

ASHTANGA YOGA

Disciple of Krishnamacharya, K. Pattabhi Jois developed the well-known ashtanga vinyasa yoga style in the twentieth century in Mysore, India. This systematic approach consists of six series, each progressively more challenging. Practitioners begin with the Primary Series, before moving to the Intermediate and Advanced Series. A key aspect of ashtanga is the *tristhana* method, which integrates breath (specifically *ujjayi*), postures, and visual gaze (*drishti*) to create a focused and transformative practice. Renowned for its progressively challenging and performative postures, the teaching methodology helps a student to cultivate self-practice. Ashtanga utilizes *surya namaskar* (sun salutation) and a fluid vinyasa application to link postures, and there is additionally a heavy emphasis on physical hands-on adjustments.

Ashtanga offers teacher-led classes where the group performs a set "series" (sequence) and is guided by the verbal instruction of an authorized teacher. More commonly, however, ashtanga provides "Mysore-style" classes, in which all students individually self-practice as the teacher moves around to offer assistance and adjustments. Mastery of the ashtanga vinyasa method requires long-term dedication and commitment to practice. The mind is able to become steady because the sequence remains the same repeatedly over a long duration of months (and sometimes years) until the student is ready to progress to the next series. Practitioners also adhere to the directive to rest on all new and full moon days plus during menstruation. All ashtanga teachers must be "authorized" or certified specifically by the institute in Mysore, most recently led by much-loved Sharath Jois, son of K. Pattabhi Jois (who has been one of multiple male teachers to come into question for inappropriate behavior toward primarily female students). With the unexpected recent passing of Sharath, the institute is now facing a new season. The rigorous and disciplined approach appeals to those seeking a physically demanding practice alongside a strong emphasis on consistency and community.

BIKRAM YOGA

The Bikram yoga style was popularized by Bikram Choudhury in the 1970s. The practice has a unique approach that includes a set sequence of twenty-six postures and two breathing exercises, always performed in a heated room. The origins of this series can be traced back to Choudhury's guru, Bishnu Charan Ghosh, as well as the influence of Bikram's own experiences with injury and illness. Choudhury drew inspiration from Hatha yoga as well as his own training as a competitive weight lifter.

The defining principles of Bikram yoga are heat, repetition, and discipline. In a typical Bikram yoga class, students practice a set sequence of postures in a room heated to 105 degrees Fahrenheit (40 degrees Celsius). The discipline required to maintain the practice in such intense conditions is regarded as an important aspect of the practice. It is claimed that the heat of the room can help the body detoxify and improve circulation, while the repetition of the set sequence allows students to gradually build strength and flexibility over time. Bikram yoga is considered to be a challenging and transformative practice that combines some traditional yoga techniques with a unique approach regarding heat and movement.

Born in 1944, Choudhury himself is no stranger to controversy. Infamous for being scantily clad and for inappropriately touching students (including, according to claims by students, sexual abuse and rape), his rise to fame and wealth eventually came crashing down. While living a lavish life of luxury, he filed for bankruptcy in 2017 after having fled the United States the year prior. In 2019 a documentary was released that detailed the rapid rise and heavy fall of his career. Despite Choudhury's reputation, Bikram yoga continues to be a popular (and at times labeled "cult-like") style of postural yoga that claims to tone and detoxify the body, relieve stress, and improve physical flexibility. Choudhury is still conducting teacher trainings annually in Thailand and is yet to be criminally prosecuted and extradited back to the United States. It is the potent practice itself that continues to draw both men and women from around the world to his signature nine-week training.

IYENGAR YOGA

Iyengar yoga is considered a precise and alignment-focused form of primarily postural yoga. It was developed by B.K.S. Iyengar, one of the most influential teachers of the twentieth century and author of multiple books. Iyengar was a student of the renowned Krishnamacharya for a brief couple of years in his youth. Born into a poor family, Iyengar suffered tremendous health issues throughout childhood. Through these challenges and his training with Krishnamacharya, he developed his signature approach. The style of Iyengar yoga emphasizes the use of props such as blocks, blankets, chairs, wall ropes, and straps to help students achieve accuracy and alignment within poses. Rarely does the approach include vinyasa-style sequencing. Instead, the postures are usually taught in a static way with longer holds, generally to promote more focused attention and awareness.

The signature emphasis on physical alignment is used initially to promote bodily awareness, strength, and mobility, but eventually also to concentrate and quieten the mind. Therefore, placing attention meticulously in and on the body is a means to encourage the practitioner to train the mind to become one-pointed. Classes often include basic pranayama techniques also. Suitable for beginners to very advanced asana practitioners, Iyengar yoga values an individualized approach where possible and has heavily influenced the development of yoga therapy and restorative yoga. Over time, through consistent practice, the technique is intended to integrate the body, mind, and emotional state.

Iyengar teacher training is different from the commonplace certification method. Teachers are required to invest in a long-term commitment to the study and training of the Iyengar methodology, similar to an apprenticeship. Once certified, there are numerous levels of accreditation to work toward over many years. With authorization to teach others, an Iyengar teacher must remain loyal to and teach only the Iyengar style and methodology. Teachers are trained thoroughly in hands-on adjustments of students, but there is also significant emphasis placed on effective verbal cueing to assist students in the attainment of postures.

KUNDALINI YOGA

"Kundalini yoga" is a term that is used across various texts and traditions. Within the context of a style of modern yoga, kundalini yoga usually relates to the style developed by Yogi Bhajan (Harbhajan Singh Puri). Originally from Punjab, in the late 1960s he took his approach from India to the global community by traveling to North America. This was a significant time, in which the popularity of yoga was increasing rapidly around the world. The Western hippie culture of the time drank up his influence and brand, which included vegetarianism, wearing white, and letting one's hair grow long. Ultimately, Yogi Bhajan's approach to yoga was a kind of fusion of Sikhism, yogic mechanics, and Tantrik teachings.

Practically speaking, a kundalini yoga practice involves a blend of mantra, kriya, postures, pranayama, and meditation. Claimed to balance the nervous and endocrine systems, the kundalini approach aims to strengthen the physical and subtle spinal column. Mantras, which are recited in the Sanskrit or Gurmukhi language, are aimed to bring about a more meditative mental state. Outwardly, kundalini yoga practitioners consume a sattvic, vegetarian diet and wear white clothing, often including a natural cloth turban or head covering. The turban is said to contain the hair—a pranic conduit—and the energy that is cultivated through the practice, with the goal of stabilizing it. The hair underneath is required to be clean, untangled, and tied up in a coiled knot. This "rishi knot," in combination with the turban, places gentle craniosacral pressure on the head around the area called the solar center.

POWER YOGA

Developed in the United States during the 1980s and 1990s, power yoga is a generally vigorous and athletic style. It was pioneered by Beryl Bender, Bryan Kest, and Baron Baptiste, each of whom studied at some point with Pattabhi Jois, founder of ashtanga yoga, among other renowned teachers. Popularized as an exercise-based practice, power yoga intends to strengthen and refine the body and mind. A typical power vinyasa yoga sequence aims to challenge and develop one's stamina, balance, flexibility, and strength. Adopted rapidly across the health and wellness industry, the methodology utilizes the vinyasa "flow" approach to linking postures and places emphasis on the engagement of ujjayi breathing.

Often performed to music, power yoga aims to synchronize movement with the breath. Props and alignment instructions are sometimes provided, but their use is minimal, generally due to the fast pace of a power yoga practice. Classes are conducted in heated studios, somewhere between 80 and 95 degrees Fahrenheit (28 to 38 degrees Celsius). Often considered to be a fitness-based workout somewhat peppered with philosophical teachings—usually from the Yoga Sutras—power yoga propagated globally in the 2000s and has, in a sense, become its own industry. Over the past two decades, power yoga studios and teachers have become synonymous with yoga apparel, brands, endorsements, and the general widespread commercialization of yoga.

RESTORATIVE YOGA

Built upon the teachings of B.K.S. Iyengar, who emphasized the use of props and modifications to support the body in various yoga postures, restorative yoga was established and refined by Judith Lasater in the 1970s. Lasater had studied directly under B.K.S. Iyengar. Naturally, restorative yoga developed out of the need for rejuvenation and restoration of the mind and body. The approach heavily uses props to support the limbs. As a result, the props facilitate the release of as much effort as possible in any posture. A full restorative practice uses fewer poses than average, each of which is held for a much longer duration. Generally, each asana is maintained for a minimum of five minutes, anywhere up to a generous twenty-minute hold. The postures are set up to be as comfortable and relaxing as possible to promote a deep sense of rest.

Activating the parasympathetic nervous system, restorative yoga is designed to feel safe, nurturing, and therapeutic, based on the interconnection of the body and mind. It uses a blend of seated, supine, and prone postures. A powerful tool for recovery and chronic stress, its slow pace can encourage the release of deeply stored tension. An accessible style of postural yoga, restorative yoga can be adapted to suit all levels of ability with the aid of blankets, blocks, bolsters, a chair, sandbags, and more. In contrast to conventional postural yoga classes, restorative yoga does not encourage any sense of stretching, tension, or collapsing. Instead, the practitioner should feel a sense of secure support—of being held—and relaxation.

SATYANANDA YOGA

Satyananda yoga is a style founded by Swami Satyananda Saraswati, a disciple of Swami Sivananda (discussed next). Reasonably, many Satyananda practitioners would argue that this is much more than a mere postural yoga style. However, Satyananda himself went on to found the Bihar School of Yoga in Munger, India, where he developed a somewhat defining approach to the practice. Anchored in the Hatha yoga tradition in union with the influence of his guru, Sivananda, Satyananda's application incorporates traditional asana (including surya namaskar), pranayama, meditation, and yoga *nidra* (usually considered a technique of yogic "sleep") alongside philosophical teachings—primarily the classical yoga of Patanjali's systematic eight-limbed approach.

The physical components of the Satyananda path include the three signature Pawanmuktasana series (joint movements), common asanas performed in a static manner, surya namaskar, shatkriya, bandha, mudra, pranayama (such as nadi shodhana), *mouna* (silence), meditation, and yoga nidra. More than a series of physical techniques and the reduction of mental suffering, Satyananda initiates follow a sattvic, vegetarian diet, partake in seva activities, recite mantras, and facilitate or participate in yajna. Satyananda centers and ashrams are spread across the globe and offer short stays, courses, and teacher trainings. Despite the abuse controversies surrounding Swami Satyananda Saraswati (who passed away in 2009), many of these centers have remained in full operation internationally, sharing his teachings and techniques. The Bihar School of Yoga has published numerous books as useful resources for practitioners and teachers. Satyananda's book, *Asana Pranayama Mudra Bandha*, is considered one of the most comprehensive yoga manuals available in print and is published in several languages.

SIVANANDA YOGA

Developed by Swami Sivananda, a renowned and respected spiritual teacher originally from Tamil Nadu, India, Sivananda yoga was further refined and propagated globally by his disciple Swami Vishnudevananda. Followed in a precise order, the Sivananda sequence involves twelve set static postures. They are designed to work together to target the entire body, to promote overall health and well-being. The signature Sivananda practice also begins with two pranayama techniques followed by surya namaskar. Shavasana is an integral component of the sequence, woven throughout as well as used at the beginning and end of the series. Overall, the full practice takes around ninety minutes.

Swami Sivananda was a medical doctor before he renounced worldly life and became a monk. He went on to become a prolific author and spiritual teacher, and his teachings continue to inspire yoga practitioners around the world today. Swami Vishnudevananda went on to found the International Sivananda Yoga Vedanta Centre's organization, a global network of Sivananda ashrams. The Sivananda school and methodology known worldwide today claims to trace through unbroken lineage back to the sage Adi Shankaracharya. The five defining principles of Sivananda yoga, as established by Vishnudevananda, are proper exercise (asana), proper breathing (pranayama), proper relaxation (shavasana), proper diet (vegetarian), and positive thinking (through the darshana of Vedanta) combined with meditation (dhyana). Anchored in Vedic teachings, the practice is designed to promote an integration of these five principles into daily life. The Sivananda approach also places emphasis on the four main paths of yoga: Karma, Bhakti, Jnana, and Raja (classical yoga).

VINIYOGA

Originally called the "viniyoga of yoga," viniyoga began as an attempt by the esteemed T.K.V. Desikachar to collate the teachings of his father, Krishnamacharya, that he received throughout the twenty-seven years of direct study with him. Intended to reflect an intelligent and systematic approach to the practice, viniyoga is aimed at a more personalized application of yoga toward any student. Suggested to be a process rather than a collection of techniques, viniyoga aspires to personalize the practice according to each individual and their circumstances, thus giving clear consideration to their age, gender, mental and physical health, lifestyle, occupation, and personal interests. Krishnamacharya instilled the belief in Desikachar that yoga should be adapted to each person, rather than making the person adapt to the practice.

Outwardly, the viniyoga approach includes slow movements with importance placed on the breath simultaneously. Function is valued over form. Postures are repeated with slow movement and also engaged in a static manner, and breath guides the poses. Other facets of yoga, such as mudra and mantra, are commonly integrated. Loosely translated to imply "appropriate application," viniyoga is more than a mere mass-marketed style of yoga. Although viniyoga does have a defining practical approach when compared to other styles of postural yoga taught across studios around the world, Desikachar's approach—and that of Krishnamacharya—was always to adapt the application of yoga to the person, and never to be branded as a style of yoga that could be taught en masse. Desikachar eventually began to separate himself from the term *viniyoga*, always preferring his original "viniyoga of yoga" and its depth of intent.

VINYASA KRAMA YOGA

Broadly applied to various applications of yoga—usually of the postural kind—the term *vinyasa krama* implies an intelligent, step-by-step progression of a sequence of actions. Therefore, vinyasa krama could apply in all sorts of non-yoga-related contexts, beyond how yogic techniques are performed. Often loosely translated as "wise progression," vinyasa krama is an intentional and mindful approach to the order of postures, actions, and practices within yoga. This includes consideration given to the gunas, the doshas, the pancha vayu, and the energetics of poses or pose categories (forward folds, backbends, inversions, twists, laterals, and so forth).

Vinyasa yoga and vinyasa krama yoga are not one and the same thing. Commonplace vinyasa yoga refers to a postural practice that links poses in a flowing manner, somewhat guided by breath. Classes can be intense (as in power yoga) or far gentler. The sequence of postures usually relates to building toward a peak pose or otherwise a particular theme or core teaching. While vinyasa krama yoga also moves in a similar manner guided by breath, the practice is always slower and guided by a different intent than mainstream vinyasa yoga.

In addition to this general approach—that is, the wise progression—there is a signature style or application of asana and pranayama in vinyasa krama that is the result of the collation of Krishnamacharya's teachings by Srivatsa Ramaswami. Ramaswami was the longest standing direct student of Krishnamacharya, other than those within his family (such as his son, T.V.K. Desikachar). He studied closely with Krishnamacharya for a period of more than three decades, which far surpasses the time that Jois or Iyengar spent with him.

Ramaswami has published multiple books and runs annual teacher trainings in India and the United States where he teaches the specific methodology he learned and systematized from the "father of modern yoga" over roughly three decades. This vinyasa krama yoga involves multiple asana sequences, each with a set focus that generally revolves around a pose category or action. Some of the asanas look more like their traditional stance (such as the "original" *trikonasana* with both feet turned outward and hips centered symmetrically). Movements are slow, calm, and breath oriented. The sequences can be basic, like the *hasta* vinyasa series—or very advanced, in a physical sense. Ramaswami's approach helps to gently develop kumbhaka and values the regular presence of pranayama. Ramaswami is rich with the knowledge of Patanjali's Yoga Sutras and recites them in Sanskrit along with other Vedic and Veda mantras. In addition, a very similar approach to the asana and pranayama of Ramaswami's vinyasa krama is taught in some kriya yoga lineages. Here the sequences are also set, the breath is lengthened, kumbhaka is cultivated, and the mind is quieted in preparation for meditation.

YIN YOGA

A modern creation based on ancient teachings, yin yoga arose from U.S. martial arts champion Paulie Zink. Regarded as a multifaceted instructor, Master Zink, who came to Hatha yoga in his early teens, is a qigong expert and a sought-after yoga teacher trainer. On the surface, Zink created the yin yoga practice—originally called Taoist yoga—as a way to mimic the poses and movements of animals to restore natural body mobility. However, at a profoundly deeper level, the practice is about working with the five elements—earth, metal, water, wood, and fire—and the energetics of the body.

The methodology arose out of Chinese Taoist principles and has been recently popularized around the world due to the work of Paul Grilley, one of Zink's students. Taking the basic elementary teachings from Zink, Grilley has since adapted and expanded upon what he learned to produce the yin yoga practiced widely in studios globally. He has amalgamated the Taoist teachings and studies with Zink with his love for anatomy and kinesiology, plus his studies with Dr. Hiroshi Motoyama.

Paul Grilley's yin yoga continues to evolve. It emphasizes the meridian theory (similar to the subtle anatomical network of nadis and marmas) and deep work with the body's connective tissue. The approach uses passive poses held for a long duration to reduce joint rigidity and congestion (the energetic kind) and untangle fascial tension. Poses are held for a minimum of three minutes and up to twenty minutes. Asymmetrical positions are usually held for less time than symmetrical ones. The majority of postures are floor based, performed seated or lying down, which supports the intent to release all muscular effort. Each student will express the poses in their own unique way due to their structural anatomy along with a sense of inner self-expression. Because of this, there is no set alignment in yin yoga.

The long-held poses apply moderate, positive stress to the ligaments, tendons, and fascia. As a result, flexibility, mobility, and circulation in the joints improve over time. In significant contrast to restorative yoga, which encourages deep relaxation and effortlessness, yin yoga moves toward an "edge" of sensation and intensity. After each posture, a short "rebound" is used to transition—often laying on the floor, as in shavasana. For the mind, yin yoga encourages the practitioner to witness their capacity to sit with and observe sensation in stillness for an extended period. Nowadays, the practice has brought in the use of props, where relevant for each individual, and the compilation of yin postures continues to grow.

Outwardly, a distinct difference between Grilley's version and the present-day yin yoga application by Paulie Zink is that Zink's style incorporates more movement and flow, with the strong influence of his extensive background and mastery in qigong. It aims to promote the mobility of Grilley's methodology but with a balance of natural strength due to the fluid movements and transitions. Both are infused with Traditional Chinese Medicine (TCM) principles and contrast with the more active, "yang" postural practices of yoga.

Four Stages of Life

Revealed through the Vedic worldview, the four stages of life, called *ashrama* (AH-shra-ma), offer any seeker a guiding framework for the broader periods of their time on earth. The ashramas are *brahmacharya*, *grhastha*, *vanaprastha*, and *sannyasa*. The way each of these life stages has been acted out over hundreds, if not thousands, of years reflects the distinct cultural context and heritage of the Indian subcontinent. While the traditional details of each stage may seem unrealistic for the average householder around the world, the essence and overarching theme of each phase is timeless in application. Commonly, the four aims of life—the aforementioned purusharthas—are loosely layered over these four stages.

In its most extreme or austere sense, the word *brahmacharya* commonly suggests the practice of sexual restraint, and it is one of the five yamas of Patanjali's eight limbs of yoga. For householders, it is more moderately considered to reflect fidelity. As it pertains to the stages of life, it is during the earlier years of the brahmacharya time when one is steeped in studentship and a restraint of indulgence in the five senses. It is the period of life to immerse in education, to cultivate discipline and establish relationships with trusted teachers or mentors. Brahmacharya is when the yamas and niyamas are instilled. Traditionally, it is the time to be anchored into the unveiling of personal dharma (the first of the purusharthas). In the present day, we could understand brahmacharya as the stage of life moving from childhood, through puberty, and into early adulthood. It is when we receive our education and ideally develop restraint from common temptations such as sexual promiscuity and the use of intoxicants. It could be regarded as a time to cultivate respect toward teachers and elders, who hold far greater wisdom and life experience. It is a time to apprentice and to refine our behavior. Brahmacharya is considered to preside over the years up until around age twenty-five. No doubt this can vary due to differences in culture and customs around the world.

Grhasta is the pivotal second phase of the average individual's life, that of the householder. Again traditionally speaking, this window of time reflects an emphasis on marriage and childbearing along with the pursuit of one's purpose, profession, and wealth of all kinds. Even without marriage or children, unless the path of renunciation is chosen, then the householder phase is inevitable for all. Often considered noble, grhasta is the period during which a spiritual path is pursued through societal duties, rather than being separate from them. Ideally, by this time dharma has been established, and thereby artha (the second purushartha) is ethically generated to support both the immediate and wider community.

As the most active of all four phases, the householder engages to serve the older and younger generations—whether directly or indirectly—through their contributions of work, wealth, and service. It is an important time to cultivate and maintain good health through self-care practices such as solid sleep, moderate sun exposure, consumption of a highly nutritional diet, good hydration, and reducing exposure to environmental toxins. Vedic texts imply that this stage of life is from approximately twenty-five years old until around age fifty. In our present-day society, given the average retirement age and extension of lifespan, this appears to extend up until around sixty-plus years old.

Vanaprastha is an initial, gentle withdrawal from society and worldly duties. In more modern or affluent terms, it could be considered "retirement." There is a consolidation of wisdom to be handed over. It is a time when responsibilities are slowly passed on to those who are younger, and the role of mentor or advisor to family and the community is taken on. Simultaneously, to some degree, it is a time to enjoy the fruits of efforts from the householder stage. The enjoyment of simple pleasures (the third purushartha, kama) is encouraged. Traditionally said to be between ages fifty and seventy-five, this life phase is a significant transition to the final time of sannyasa.

Vanaprastha is a step into a peripheral role that focuses on service and spiritual pursuits. There is a detachment from economic or wealth-generation roles and, ideally, a renewed care for the state of society and the environment that will be left behind. Most often, those in this latter stage of life reflect a wisdom from their lived experiences and relinquishment of material attachments or gains. Life becomes more simplified and reflective. One's finances are (hopefully) in order. Pleasure and joy are found in the seemingly ordinary. Throughout history and the Vedic worldview, vanaprastha also has been a literal withdrawal to the edges of society, to be a forest-dweller and prepare for the final years.

Sannyasa is the final and fourth of the ashramas, that of renunciation. It is the stage of life where the yogic practices and teachings culminate and are inherently reflected through embodiment. This time is seen as a last opportunity to resolve or fulfill any remaining karma. This could be through the resolution of practical duties such as conflicts, debts, or unfulfilled aspects of the individual dharma. Alternatively, it could be through ardent spiritual sadhana. Directly related to the fourth of the purusharthas, moksha, the sannyasa years are the transitional portal when impending death is at the forefront. Unless householder life was renounced entirely—in the case of monks and sadhus, for example, who move from brahmacharya to sannyasa—it is finally a complete withdrawal from the material desires and possessions. Sadly, in our present-day world we see many at the end of life intensely clinging to their youth or physical belongings. Traditionally, the renunciant phase inspires an immense simplification within every aspect of life. Ideally, actions are oriented inward, food consumption is minimal, and the mind is unburdened by societal stress. Ultimately, one's quality of life during sannyasa reflects choices made throughout earlier years.

An appreciation of the four ashramas gives us a broader perspective on the trajectory of life. Awareness of each stage can refine our values and inform our choices throughout the day-to-day. *Ashrama dharma* is a term used for the specific duties or general roles within each of the four phases. In earlier times, this was also shaped by caste, gender, and marital status, not only age. The Vedic vision of the ashrama helps us to zoom out and have reverence for the bigger picture and purpose of each meaningful life phase. These guidelines are timeless and adaptable toward the continued evolution of society and culture around the world.

Ayurvedic Stages of Life

Fundamentally founded upon the five elements of nature (space, air, fire, water, and earth) that make up the macrocosm and microcosm, Ayurveda seeks to bring each individual into harmony with their environment. This includes all the seasons and transitions across a lifespan, from birth to death. These five elements join together in combinations to create the three doshas: *vata*, *pitta*, and *kapha*. Vata consists of air and space, pitta consists of fire and water, and kapha consists of water and earth.

The three doshas in various ratios are inherently a part of all human beings, depending on our genetics and circumstances. The qualities of these three doshas govern different periods of any twenty-four-hour cycle: vata governs the window of 2 a.m. to 6 a.m. and 2 p.m. to 6 p.m.; pitta rules 10 a.m. to 2 p.m. and 10 p.m. to 2 a.m.; and kapha dominates from 6 a.m. to 10 a.m. and 6 p.m. to 10 p.m. In addition, the three doshas—and their qualities—govern the changing seasons of each year, the climate of each day, and also the broader stages of life.

Ayurveda has its origins within the Vedas, specifically the Rigveda and Atharvaveda. This *upaveda* (subveda) is intrinsically connected to the yogic traditions and culture of certain parts of the Indian subcontinent. Some would suggest that to truly *live* yoga, one must be steeped in the essence of Ayurveda as a minimum.

Through the Ayurvedic lens, the average lifespan is divided into roughly three phases, each of which is governed by one of the doshas. The qualities that characterize each of the doshas are physiologically increased during their distinctive stage of life. Importantly, our own constitution (usually called *prakriti*) and current state (*vikruti*) are always significant when pursuing specific health outcomes or understanding best lifestyle practices. However, similar to the aforementioned stages of life as per the general Vedic worldview, these elemental qualities fundamentally correlate with various physiological states and changes in the human body (and mind). There is no defining moment when we move from one phase to the next. Instead, there is a natural and gradual transition, during which the body is required to adapt and adjust. Certain qualities are increased as others decrease. Any physical or mental health issues, mild or severe, are usually reflective of an excess dominance of any one of the doshas over time. Despite the noteworthy differences between individuals and their unique circumstances, to have awareness of how the doshas preside over these three major seasons of a person's lifetime helps any individual take proactive steps to experience greater attunement and alignment with the innate rhythms of life.

Kapha dominates the first of the three Ayurvedic life stages. Conception is the start of this particular phase, and it ends around the time puberty begins. Therefore, the kapha stage overlaps the earlier part of the brahmacharya time. The earth and water elements of kapha are reflected in qualities that are heavy, cool, stable, soft, dense, and slow. Within the physiology, kapha relates to the functions of building structure, growth, nourishment, hydration or lubrication, and cohesion. Kapha supports anabolic processes. This is all demonstrated through the growth of a baby through their infancy and into childhood. Cells continuously generate; body mass increases significantly; new tissues are built; the skin, hair, and eyes are lustrous; fat is used as fuel; and love and affection are regularly emanated, while sweet and fatty foods are favored. With an excess of kapha, children can be prone to congestion, runny noses, coughs, asthma, and more.

Pitta governs the second phase of life, according to Ayurveda. Made up of fire and water, this dosha presides over the longest period, starting from puberty and continuing until around age fifty to fifty-five. Over these years the pitta qualities that increase are understood to be hot, sharp, light, oily, spreading, and subtle. Pitta manages the physiological functions of transformation, digestion, assimilation, and temperature regulation. Throughout this time, we witness more heat in the body, which manifests in various symptoms—think of the impacts of puberty or of menopause on the body and mind, for example.

Pitta is inherently fiery. In excess, it can promote imbalances that may lead to inflammation, skin conditions, eye issues, hyperacidity, heartburn, hormonal imbalance, IBS, acne, anger, impatience, and irritability.

In a more positive sense, pitta inspires drive and ignites ambition, discipline, and dedication. It therefore relates to the latter stage of brahmacharya and supports the many grhastha years of the householder. We can embrace and utilize the positive pitta qualities to remain motivated, physically active, and mentally sharp. Keep in mind that if pitta is aggravated over the long term and during the latter years, it has a detrimental ripple effect that flows into the final Ayurvedic stage of life. Literally and figuratively, we end up burnt out from the fire and are left with a dry, barren physical and mental vessel.

Vata presides over the final phase of the Ayurvedic life cycle. Approximately from age fifty or fifty-five until death, air and space reign. The body and mind reflect the distinct qualities of vata, that which is cold, dry, rough, mobile, and light. Generally, the vata dosha relates to movement of all kinds—physical but also mental—as well as creativity, expansiveness, and communication. Throughout these years, the body dries up the reservoir of youth, and softness, immunity, and strength diminish. Usually a gradual depletion is experienced.

These elder years of vata dominance generally correspond to the vanaprastha and sannyasa stages of life. If an individual has overdone the previous period governed by pitta, this latter phase can send them into rapid decline. The skin dries up, bone and muscle deteriorate, the digestive functions slow down significantly, the mind dulls, joint pain increases, and potentially devastating conditions become apparent (consider those living with Alzheimer's or Parkinson's disease). This stage of life, according to Ayurveda, requires warmth, lubrication (externally on the skin and also internally through hydrating food choices), rest, reflection, and stability. In the most positive sense, the vata years have the potential to be experienced as full of creativity, wisdom, deep spiritual inquiry, satisfaction, and quietude. If the focus is on nourishment and simplification—on all levels—then the process of a peaceful withdrawal from worldly duties and desires becomes entirely natural. Unfortunately, society is currently set up to induce depletion and burnout for most.

Harnessing the wisdom of Ayurveda to embrace its fundamental principles ensures that life can be lived far more smoothly and harmoniously. The Ayurvedic framework of the three stages loosely overlapped upon the traditional four ashramas (which the four purushartha are woven into) can strengthen our yogic pursuits. To adjust and direct

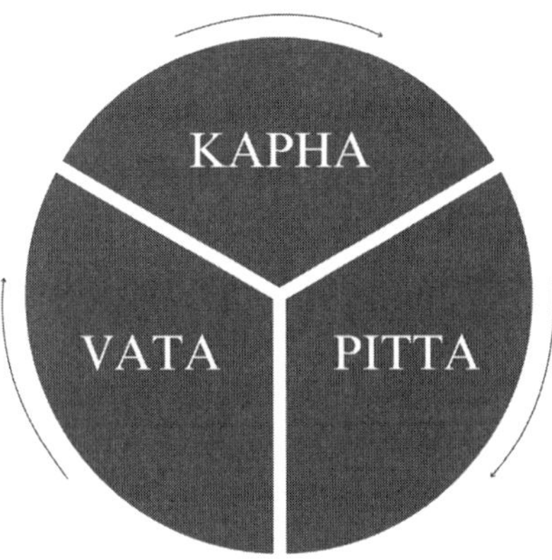

FIGURE 5. The three ayurvedic doshas that govern various aspects of the cycles and rhythms of life

choices, actions, and duties with these understandings shifts yoga from an exclusively isolated practice to something that is genuinely lived. It also encourages a greater sense of trust and surrender toward the unfoldment of daily life.

How Many Limbs?

In Sanskrit, a common translation of *anga* (AH-nga) relates to the physical body. More specifically, it speaks to the various literal limbs (head, hands, waist, feet, and so on), which are seen across many of the Indian dance traditions. This includes the more minor limbs, called *pratyangas* and *upangas*. Across these dance forms, the limbs are used to express certain gestures, called *angika-abhinaya*, as taught in the esteemed *Natya Shastra* text.

Perhaps a more well-known use of *anga* is through the translation "subdivision." Patanjali's ashtanga approach refers to eight divisions, or limbs, of the path. We could say that these are eight aids that together compound over time to move us toward the state of yoga. Given the popularity of Patanjali's teachings, it is common for students of yoga to assume that there are eight definitive limbs across all traditions. But how many limbs are there really? Which limbs are deemed more superior? Do the limbs vary in their order and application? As is often the case, the answer depends on the text and the tradition.

While Patanjali teaches of the eight limbs of yoga, there are further, prominent auxiliaries from other renowned masters and within revered texts. These *yoganga* are often offered in a sequential manner, like the limbs of Patanjali's ashtanga yoga. For example, the *shadanga* (six-limbed) yoga taught across Hatha and Tantrik texts is made up of asana, pranayama, pratyahara, dharana, dhyana, and samadhi. The yamas and niyamas are omitted, but not because they are of no importance. On the contrary, they are assumed to be foundational and thereby already integrated and embodied. In the shadanga approach, other techniques are regarded as important further divisions that relate to asana (similar to the yamas and niyamas being made up of multiple applications). Those are usually mudra, bandha, and the *shatchakra* (which are not given significance in Patanjali's ashtanga).

Across the broad yoga traditions and varied texts, there can be four, five, six, seven, eight, and even fifteen limbs. Within this diversity, there is one limb that appears to have consistent significance, not to mention a timeless relevance. In Sanskrit it is called *tarka*. More commonly translated as "reasoning" and "inquiry," tarka suggests a high level of discernment. Without a fall into cynicism, tarka inspires a sense of reasonable doubt and questioning with the ultimate goal of uncovering the truth. Importantly, it requires a sense of emotional composure and neutrality. Tarka is not attained through suspicion, aversion, or criticism for the aim of satisfying one's own beliefs. Tarka arises out of the quest to refine knowledge.

The praised North Indian polymath, Abhinavagupta—a mystic, philosopher, aesthetician, and theologian—pressed that tarka was the most supreme of all limbs on the path. He believed this highest insight through acute discernment, called *sat-tarka*, is the most direct means to the attainment of yoga. Considered a Tantrik master, Abhinavagupta greatly influenced the various schools of Tantra and described a six-limbed path. However, this shadanga approach is that of the *trika* yoga of Kashmir Shaivism, where the six auxiliaries are pranayama (including kumbhaka), dharana, tarka, dhyana, samadhi, and pratyahara (as absorption of the mind).

In addition, many schools of Indian philosophical teachings speak to the value of tarka and its place in debate and discussion. In a far more exalted manner, tarka is also considered as a shastra, or treatise. *Tarkashastra* encompasses an entire systematic philosophical approach to logic, reasoning, and the art of debate that may involve relentless questioning until a truth is distilled. The goal is attainment of the highest knowledge, for the good of all.

The diversity of the Indian subcontinent is reflected in the diversity of yoga. There are many varied steps and paths to the destination. Ultimately, any limb mentioned within the yogic traditions will likely not result in realization of the goal if applied in isolation. Over-intellectualization of each can be a hinderance on the path also. However, there is no doubt that some of the limbs are more highly regarded due to their effectiveness and potency. *Bhavana* (sometimes called *bhava*) is a limb that, in this context, refers to "attitude." For householders on the path, this auxiliary has profound importance. In the least, any embodied attitude toward dharma, spiritual pursuits, wise counsel of teachers, community, and yogic texts and traditions plays a role in the resolution—or cultivation—of karma and samskaras.

Philosophical Systems

A risk of speaking to the numerous "philosophical systems" that have arisen out of the Indian subcontinent is the implication that the teachings become easily compartmentalized, which in reality is not the case. There is always a cross-pollination of ideas and beliefs, even while notable differences are upheld. The English term "philosophy" can lead one down an impersonal, theoretical, and overly academic path—which is no issue if that is your intention. For practitioners, however, these systems are best observed and learned as teachings that are rich, poetic, relational, alive, and lived—not simply discussed or studied. It is also important to note, not all philosophical teachings emerge out of the Vedas (as in the case of Buddhist and Jain yoga). Nor is Sanskrit the only language of yogic philosophy and texts.

To unpack these teachings, a combined analytical and tangible approach is required. Fundamentally, the multiple philosophical systems do not merely intersect with yogic techniques and practicalities; they are considered inseparable. However, their transformational relevance can seem elusive if not studied in depth with a genuine authority: that is, a masterful teacher who has longstanding embodiment, who is a genuine steward. These teachings are intended to support the cultivation of a yogic lifestyle, living and breathing a particular tradition. To study any philosophical shastra systematically with a teacher, and simultaneously patiently apply the knowledge, has the potential to alleviate a wealth of suffering on the path. This intentional approach to studentship inspires growth and smarana (self-remembrance). Each sampradaya will have specified texts to repeatedly return to. A commitment to studying yogic teachings of any kind is to delve into an array of subjects that are not only considered ancient, but that are layered, applicable, accessible (for the most part), and yet complex at times. Yoga "philosophy"—a construct of the Western language—is both broad and deep. To appreciate this vastness is to keep the mind open, curious, and discerning.

Darshana is a Sanskrit word often used for various schools of thought. For example, Patanjali's classical yoga is considered a darshana. *Darshana* usually translates to "perceive," "behold," or "see." The essence of darshana is inextricably woven into daily life in India, as when one visits a temple and receives an auspicious glimpse of the deity. As it relates to the philosophical traditions, darshana can refer to shastra. Alternatively, it suggests contemplation, examination, experience, virtue, knowledge, attainment of perspective, and noticing or demonstrating. Darshana is imbued with the essence of reverence and humility. Thus, while lesser known globally, it is a far better word (as shastra can be also) to describe the numerous schools of thought or belief—some of which are considered heterodox (*nastika*) and others orthodox (*astika*). Again, these are Western constructs that can be limiting. Sometimes contested, the most common distinction is that the orthodox schools such as Vedanta see the Vedas as the authority. Heterodox schools, like Jainism, do not.

Grouped together, the *shad-darshana* are the six major astika schools of thought. These are Samkhya, Yoga, Nyayah, Mimamsa, Vaisheshika, and Vedanta. Of these, Samkhya, Yoga, and Vedanta appear to have the greatest influence on the yogic teachings and techniques that have proliferated in recent decades. Founded by the sage Kapila, Samkhya is generally considered dualistic, as it makes a distinction between *purusha* (spirit, or consciousness) and prakriti (matter, or the manifest). The Sanskrit word *samkhya*, depending on the context, is usually translated as "enumerate," "calculate," "reason," or "deliberate." The Samkhya school lays forth the twenty-five *tattvas* (principles) and the three gunas of sattva, rajas, and tamas. Purusha is one of the twenty-five principles, with the other twenty-four being aspects of reality or the manifest world, from subtle to gross. This categorization of the cosmos is a reflection of the theoretical and metaphysical emphasis within Samkhya. The foundational and oldest surviving text of this darshana is the *Samkhyakarika*. There is also a suggestion that Kapila and his agnostic Samkhya shastra influenced some Buddhist traditions.

With certainty, the school of classical yoga adopted the systematic Samkhya theory of the twenty-five tattvas and the three gunas. Monotheistic and considered dualistic (although sometimes disputed), this darshana was founded by the sage Patanjali. Not to be confused with the broader term of "yoga," this classical approach is practically reflected in the well-known eightfold path of ashtanga yoga (as per Patanjali's Yoga Sutras, which is the foundational text of this school of thought); that being yama, niyama, asana, pranayama, pratyahara, dharana, dhyana, and samadhi. Patanjali's yoga is no doubt a more practical and technical system—comparative to samkhya—that places value on meditation, ethics, and discipline.

The Yoga Yajnavalkya is considered another important text that endorses the classical yoga tradition. Both the Yoga and Samkhya darshanas consider there to be only three means (*pramana*) to valid knowledge, and they are *pratyaksha* (perception), *anumana* (inference), and *shabda* (testimony from a reliable source). Many would fairly suggest that Samkhya and Yoga appear one and the same (or, at least that they were initially), given the dualistic approach of each.

Perhaps even more relevant to the yoga we know today, Vedanta is primarily nondualistic and founded upon the knowledge of the Upanishads and Brahma Sutras. There are a number of subtraditions in Vedanta (including a dualistic one called Dvaita), perhaps the most common of which is Advaita Vedanta, expounded by scholar and renowned acharya Adi Shankara along with others. The *jivanmukta* Ramana Maharishi reflected much of the Advaita wisdom through his advocacy of introspective self-inquiry, Jnana and Bhakti yoga, universal oneness of consciousness, and more. In addition, the essence of the Upanishads—and more specifically Advaita Vedanta—is revealed through the Mahavakyas, the "great sayings." The most common of these expressions or tenets is *tat tvam asi* (meaning "thou art that") and *aham Brahmasmi* (meaning "I am Brahman" or "I am the Supreme divinity").

Also called Uttara Mimamsa (implying "latter inquiry"), Vedanta concerns itself with rumination on the supreme universal principle of Brahman. It also values examination of the eternal consciousness that resides within each individual, called Atman. Across all of the Vedanta traditions, shastra is regarded as being the highest and most reliable source of knowledge. Hence there are many commentaries that expound the core Vedantic ideas found within the various Upanishads and especially the Bhagavad Gita. Revealed scripture is deemed the authority. Common concepts such as karma, samsara, and *maya* (usually referring to "illusion" or that which conceals reality and truth) are upheld across the Vedantic teachings. However, they may be understood in contrasting ways across the different traditions. There is a devotional thread through most, if not all, of the subschools of Vedanta. Experiential perception and inference are also considered essential on the path.

While each of the subschools of Vedanta hold their own distinctions—and deserve a wealth of study, time, and contemplation beyond the scope of this book—at the heart of it, Vedanta promotes a reverence that at the very least inspires a unifying attitude toward all. An astonishingly beautiful text that conveys the essence of Advaita Vedanta is the *Ashtavakra Gita*. Originally presented as a dialogue between King Janaka and the sage Ashtavakra, each passage aims toward Self-realization. An example of this is through the simple yet profound words of sutra 2.10:

> MATTO VINIRGATAM VISHVAM MAYYEVA LAYAMESHYATI |
> MRDI KUMBHO JALE VICIH KANAKE KATAKAM YATHA || 2.10 ||
>
> *From me the world streams out*
> *And in me it dissolves,*
> *As a bracelet melts into gold,*
> *A pot crumbles into clay,*
> *A wave subsides in water.*[9]

Over the past centuries, Tantra has greatly influenced the yoga that is now regularly practiced around the world. Often misinterpreted and therefore misrepresented, the subject of Tantra is a mammoth one. The word *tantra*, in a broad context, can relate to texts (like the *Tantras*) or a methodology, theory, teaching, technique, or instrument. In Sanskrit, *tantra* means "loom" or "warp." Usually considered heterodox, Tantra has many subtraditions—some dualistic but mostly nondual. The root word *tan* means "weave," "to extend," or "put forth." *Tra* means "instrument." This suggests that the word *tantra* can imply a doctrine, science, or system to be shared.

Rather than the Vedas being the primary authority, the Agamas (AH-gamas) are the major collection of literature that Tantra is founded upon and are written in Sanskrit and Tamil. While the goal of Tantra may be Self-realization, the nondualistic Tantra simultaneously cherishes the material world of existence. It reveres all of nature, such as the microcosmic human form and the five elements. Therefore, it could be considered an incredibly relevant and practical path for the average householder. In Tantra, instead of promoting disidentification with the body, the teachings and techniques advocate for going *through* the body to go beyond the body.

In the Western world, Tantra is often synonymous with messages of "sacred sex" via New Age Tantra or Neo-Tantra, which is often an approach devoid of other essential facets of a Tantrik path. Even across the Indian subcontinent, Tantra is usually perceived as some kind of black magic or occultism. The reality is that, while some of the Tantrik traditions do include the use of intoxicants, consumption of meat, and an engagement in sexual practices (such as retention of sexual fluids) during rituals, these are far less common and are reserved for advanced practitioners. The reason is that they can be addictive and reinforce attachments to sensory pleasure and enjoyment. Some more common characteristics of a Tantrik path are techniques that—moving toward entrainment—use awareness, visualization, pranayama, mudra, bandha, mantra, and more.

Like other paths, Tantrik practitioners place great value on the authority of the guru or teacher. Sincere practitioners are initiated into a specific subtradition, for most of the techniques are *rahasya*—closely guarded and kept secret, away from the eyes and ears of the uninitiated. Symbolism, such as yantra, mandala, or chakra (the choice generally depends on the tradition) is used within rituals.

It is suggested that Tantra is potentially much older than originally thought, and that Tantra may have actually informed the Vedas and classical yoga. There is also speculation that perhaps Patanjali was in fact a Tantrik practitioner. What is for certain is that current-day yoga can be traced back to the Hatha yoga tradition, and this Hatha yoga tradition is traced back to *classical* Tantra. Classical Tantra, also known as Shaivism, had a tremendous influence on the development of a Buddhist path known as Vajrayana along with Tibetan Buddhism. One of the most well-known strands of Shaivism is Kashmir Shaivism, which was deeply influenced by the work of Abhinavagupta, namely his treatise called the *Tantraloka.* Perhaps one of the most studied texts of Kashmir Shaivism is the *Vijnana Bhairava Tantra*, written sometime between the seventh and eighth century and a sacred scripture of the nondualistic Kaula Trika sampradaya. Historically, some form of Tantra (mostly Shaivism) propagated across the Indian subcontinent and even across to Indonesia.

Generally speaking, Tantra is considered theistic and mostly non-dual and arose out of the esoteric *agamic* texts called the Tantras. The broad tradition involves anthropomorphic worship of divinity. It embraces both internal ritual (*antaryaga*) and external ritual (*bahiryaga*). An example of this is the installment and worship of an internally cultivated or external physical yantra, such as the Sri Chakra. Another example is the worship of the internal subtle fire and the external fire, as in puja or yajna. Entirely contrasted to the kundalini yoga of Yogi Bhajan, the term "kundalini yoga" arises in Tantra traditions also, due to the techniques and attention placed on the subtle pranic anatomy, namely working with the chakras, bindu, kundalini arousal, and beyond.

One of the most renowned Tantrik traditions is that of Shri Vidya. This is a *shakta* or Devi-focused path that honors and worships the goddess, the divine feminine. At the heart of it, Shri Vidya is an intimacy with and celebration of the goddess Lalita Tripura Sundari and the great universal cosmic power. In the Tantrik goddess traditions generally, Shakti is regarded as being both unmanifest consciousness *and* energy. She is upheld in the prominent role of Supreme creator and what has been created. She is the source and the substance of all things. This is in contrast to the Tantrik traditions where the male deity—Shiva—is the universal consciousness, and Devi is his consort of creative capacity who manifests through him. Across the Shakti traditions there are many subschools with various goddesses of worship at the forefront. The most popular texts of study for aspirants immersed in Devi worship are the

Lalita Sahasranama, *Saundarya Lahari*, *Devi Bhagavata Purana*, and the revered *Devi Mahatmya*.

The wealth of revered Tantrik texts across all traditions are at times intentionally elusive, vague, and mystical in their teachings. This is due to the expectation that the finer details of techniques are passed on through oral tradition by the guru or initiated (and competent) practitioner. In Tantra broadly speaking, every thing and every experience in life holds juice to be extracted out of it. Everything is to be embraced—the good, the bad, and the ugly, so to speak—and is seen as a potential tool for liberation. There is no material renunciation to be pursued. Everything is divine. Even a dense rock is an expression of Shiva. All aspects of nature are deeply sacred.

There is an extraordinary diversity of traditions that have arisen out of the Indian subcontinent, highlighting the multitude of paths one has the potential to navigate. The beauty in this is that it reflects a long-standing tolerance of and open-mindedness about different perspectives and applications of transformative knowledge that lead toward a similar goal or vision. Each path offers the potential to understand our reality—and what is beyond it—in a way that provides spiritual nourishment and also a deep respect for time-tested wisdom. There is an ocean of possibility available to any sincere seeker. However, this can potentially stir up a sense of overwhelm. With this, it is to be remembered that there is no need for—nor any benefit in—gathering information on many of these varied traditions. This would be intellectualization and mental accumulation. The broad overview offered here is to merely provide some simple, comparative perspective. Furthermore, it hopefully instills a greater sense of alignment with one particular direction to pursue in depth (and ideally with the guidance of an embodied teacher).

On Teaching Yoga

What does it mean to be a *teacher* of yoga? How has the title of "yoga teacher" shifted? What is it that qualifies a person to teach? What indicates success as a yoga teacher? These are all important questions that hold answers with immense nuance. Every year in the United States, thousands of people get certified in the framework of a 200-hour teacher training program. The older model of apprenticeship is all but lost. Around the world, there is a widespread disconnection from the cultural context of yoga and therefore repeated instances of misappropriation. This is not to be conflated with a natural appropriation that arises due to the integration of various cultures and communities slowly over time through the exchange of ideas.

Most would likely agree that the majority of folks teaching yoga are postural yoga *instructors*. The title of "instructor" holds a subtle yet powerful distinction from "teacher," despite their being used interchangeably. (They are synonyms, after all.) An instructor instructs; they *tell* people what to *do*. This could be considered a more mechanical role, and one that is easy to replicate (as reflected in almost all teacher training programs). A teacher *teaches*. Instruction is certainly a *part* of what they do, but a teacher aims to guide and transform others on a deeper level. A teacher's knowledge and experience are not as easy to duplicate or imitate. These qualities reflect years of embodiment. Consider the skill and knowledge required to teach someone how to handcraft high-quality furniture that will last lifetimes, for example. Then compare this with a manual with instructions on how to build a piece of flat-pack furniture. Both methods of communicating how to build do serve in some way. They have practical, beneficial outcomes, but to different degrees, with vastly different results. Within the context of yoga, this distinction alludes to the tremendous value of studentship.

To confidently uphold integrity as a yoga *teacher*, and to become an effective channel for transmission, one must be steeped in continuous commitment to one's role as a student. This is not to point toward accumulating knowledge or certifications, even though these are no doubt helpful to a degree, on the surface level. Instead, this intent requires a long-term dedication to the yogic vision and the assimilation of, reflection on, and repeated marination in the teachings. All this is to be held with both great trust and patience.

A teacher shares from the heart, from wisdom, experience, and inherent self-worth. An instructor is more inclined to share from the training handbook—that is, things intellectually learned from a course or program that still need more time to be assimilated and lived. This distinction is not meant to evoke cynicism. Both roles offer value and are needed in society. Rather, it is to create clarity through discernment so that each person—whether student or teacher—can come to understand their role in stewardship and the continued evolution of yoga, within their community and across the globe at large.

In the Vedic tradition, a student takes at least twelve years—one cycle of Jupiter—to learn something before they are considered eligible to share with others, then the guru must give their blessing first. This is not to imply that a yoga teacher should or needs to teach everything they learn, such as a full spectrum of yogic techniques, texts, and philosophical teachings. Rather, it suggests that being immersed in a well-rounded path of personal practice can bear fruits that create a higher level of discernment and clarity about what to share and what to keep closely guarded. A breadth of knowledge and understanding offers anyone on the path the foundational insight on how to engage with yoga as a *way of life*. This could come through complementary studies in Ayurveda, Jyotisha, Vastu, or Indian martial forms, for example.

The wider the field of study, the more evident it becomes how all the rich traditions of the Indian subcontinent are inextricably woven together and further strengthened in unison. But again, all these facets of Indic culture do not need to be taught to students. In fact, in most cases, this would be overwhelming, especially without a thorough foundational context for the student. This reinforces the validity of a teacher having invested in their fields of study for a lengthy period of time so they can sincerely grasp what and how the knowledge needs to be communicated—a process that is always slower than expected (or hoped).

It is through this extensive immersion, maturation, and deepening of personal experience that a yoga teacher comes to know what is appropriate (and thereby ethical) to impart to any student or within their community. While it is true that teaching others what we know helps us to further embody the knowledge, not everything learned needs to be taught. Of even more importance is the teacher's acknowledgment of what the student is best suited to receive, given that person's level of knowledge, studentship, and dedication. And it may not always be what the student desires! The teacher offers enrichment through the upliftment of knowledge *and* upholding boundaries—that is, what the ideal information (posture, practice, guidance) is to be delivered and at what ideal time. In the modern world, the tendency for humankind is to want to learn something fast and on-demand at any moment desired. The yoga tradition has never operated in this way (until recently). Reflected throughout centuries in India, whether one is a student of a strand of yoga, classical music, dance, sculpting, carving, or weaving, the teacher *very* slowly (and sometimes cryptically!) offers guidance or instruction. The student is expected to repeat, repeat, repeat what has been taught to them, hundreds if not thousands of times over. Patience is a crucial prerequisite. Then, the teacher decides what and how much it is apt to impart next. There is a magnificent lesson in this.

Mastery of the highest knowledge takes years before it becomes wisdom and is embodied in every cell. No doubt this realization could derail someone who is aspiring to teach yoga. Alternatively, it could inspire a wholehearted, lifelong commitment. Therefore, it is imperative to uncover the motivation to pursue yoga teaching or instruction. For many, it arises from a life-changing experience with yoga that creates a strong yearning to share it with others. For some, the yoga practice offers solace from the hardships of daily life. For others the pursuit of teaching can be an escape from an existing career path that presents a lack of fulfillment. The path of a yoga teacher can be alluring. However, does the desire correspond to a person's dharma?

Significantly, popularity as a teacher does not automatically equate to expertise. This is a grand misconception due to the rise of social media. Many masterful teachers completely shy away from the online world, but it is a real balancing act for yoga teachers of today who wish to be of service, honor the source of the teachings, and also need to pay the bills. Most yoga teachers are householders, and the cultivation of artha (wealth) through dharma is a fundamental part of life, according to the Vedic worldview. Through an alluring pursuit that ensures basic needs are met, when life can be enjoyed (adherence to kama) and an overall sense of financial security is ever-present, there is still a risk of straying away from the inner compass of integrity. This might look like teaching an excessive number of classes to gain popularity or income and, as a result, losing one's personal practice. It may look like accepting opportunities to teach that are paid poorly or honoring a request to present yoga in a way that is out of alignment with one's approach and qualifications. It could be time constraints that inhibit a teacher's capacity to take students into deeper realms of practice that they may be seeking (whether consciously or not). It may look like teaching outside of one's scope of practice instead of referring students on to someone with more experience. There is no doubt that the rapid commercialization of yoga has contributed to, if not caused, these challenges.

Yoga teaching can come with other struggles that have the potential to poorly impact mental health. These may include the experience of workplace politics and abuse, favoritism, or doing excess amounts of unpaid labor. It could also be a dependency on the title and role of a yoga teacher to gain external validation. This only results in disillusionment and an dependency on (positive) feedback from students and peers. If a yoga teacher repeatedly compromises their intrinsic sense of integrity to serve the demands of students or studio owners, the outcome is immense exhaustion at the least. All is not lost, however. A sense of self-worth can be derived from a dedication to studentship. This generates an overflow of inspiration, clarity, and creativity. When there is a long-term vision and commitment to the path, it is easier to feel less hurried to achieve a certain perception of success. In turn, students are provided a grounded foundation that fosters a steady growth and glorious depth on their journey.

Swami Kuvalayananda gave us some pertinent words to contemplate: "Yoga should not be diluted." With this front of mind, teachers are forced to consider their responsibilities around cultural relevance and how to uphold yogic principles within a capitalist society. Ethics play a huge part in teaching yoga effectively and respectfully. Within the context of yoga teaching, professional ethics are not confined to yamas and niyamas. Yoga teachers have a duty to be well versed in their responsibilities toward student safety, teacher–student relations, physical adjustments, appropriate dress, liabilities, language and communication (Sanskrit is too often shunned in studio classes and profanities celebrated!), scope of practice, confidentiality, general legalities, business, accounting, marketing, equity of opportunity, source-culture awareness, cultural context, and more. These are all components of the professional path for a yoga teacher, though they are beyond the scope of this book. Donna Farhi, a senior teacher from New Zealand, does offer "practical and provocative" insight in her book *Teaching Yoga*. In part one, as she explores the sacred role of the teacher, Farhi proposes the question, "What is a yoga teacher?" She goes on:

> Yoga is not simply information that the teacher carries and disseminates separate from herself, to be left in the classroom or studio at the end of the workday. What is being taught is a state of being, a way of living, which by necessity is intrinsic to the character of the teacher. In the study of Yoga, the teacher can lead the student only as far as she has gone herself. She can empathize with the student's spiritual quest, and the issues that may arise during that quest, only because she herself has embarked on such a journey. For this reason, it is difficult to separate the professional life from the personal life of a Yoga teacher. How can a way of life and a state of being be turned on and off at whim or divested when it is convenient to do so?[10]

An effective yoga teacher demonstrates what it is to weave yoga throughout daily life. This is reflected through their deep connection to the practice and therefore conveyed through how they share the transformative potency of yoga with sincerity, even within the framework of a sixty-minute class. There is an essence of integrity that is imbibed, and the goal or vision of the teacher puts the teachings, the tradition, and the student's experience at the forefront.

In bringing this reflective section on teaching yoga to a close, the following passage from the Upadeshasahasri holds nectar for a yoga teacher to contemplate:

> The teacher is the one who can see a question from both sides and has memory. The teacher is endowed with tranquility, self-control, compassion, skill, and the desire to help others. The teacher is versed in sacred and traditional knowledge and is well established in those teachings. The teacher maintains integrity and is free from self-interest, arrogance, boastfulness, obsession and deception. Such a teacher's only aim is to transmit knowledge and thus relates to the student clearly and fondly.[11]

CONTEMPLATIONS

What is my relationship with the guru principle, or the role of the guru, and why?

What stage of life am I in right now, through the Vedic lens and an Ayurvedic perspective?

Knowing this, how can I make adjustments to further embody yoga throughout my daily life?

Which of the numerous yogic traditions do I feel the deepest resonance with and why?

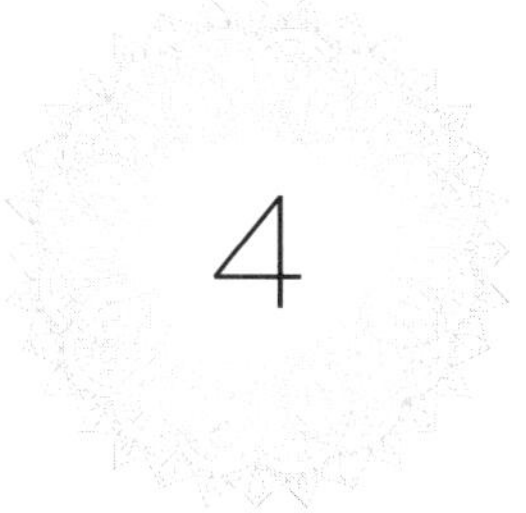

INWARD

A PRACTICAL FRAMEWORK

IN AN EFFORT TO COUNTER the intellectual considerations that have been presented thus far, it is crucial to outline the potential practical way inward. To read and listen to information without application leaves yoga to be experienced through the outer mind only. However, yoga cannot be truly understood intellectually. It must be engaged with so that interiorization is not just an idea, but cultivated and sustained directly. This message has been beautifully articulated by German Canadian Indologist and yoga scholar Georg Feuerstein:

> Even if we read a thousand books on oceanography or on maritime adventures, we cannot really understand the ocean unless we jump into the water ourselves and get wet . . . The situation is similar in regard to the ocean of Yoga. We can learn many facts about Yoga, but they will give us only an external view of it. In order to truly understand Yoga, we must engage its living reality and allow it to teach us.[12]

Components of a Complete Practice

What are the aspects of a yoga practice that make it whole and balanced? What are the elements that reflect yoga as a path beyond the postures? How does a practice reflect abhyasa? What is it that makes a sadhana effective?

A yogic journey, in its truest sense, inspires a letting go of self-identification. It is one that reflects a progressive interiorization, one that infiltrates all aspects of our life. Slowly, our practice ideally unveils our highest state and reveals the reality of who we inherently are. But how do we get there?

This section of the book aims to serve the yearning for a more wholesome, holistic experience that is founded in a broad and traditional approach. That is not to suggest that everything presented here must be utilized, and certainly not all at once. However, it is useful to inquire into the numerous components that can contribute to a far more effective grounding in yoga. When we consider the more tangible techniques of yoga, they can be likened to a tapestry. Weaving the various sacred threads together allows our efforts to feel far more cohesive and cumulative.

The term *sarvanga sadhana* implies a personal yoga practice that is thoughtfully well rounded and inclusive of the many fibers that strengthen our embodiment of yoga (weaving our own tapestry). The word *sarvanga* refers to "all limbs" or "whole body." On the most superficial level, this is an invitation to see yoga beyond the asana. That is not to suggest any removal or omission of physical postures. Quite the contrary. By embracing other facets of yoga, we can deepen and enrich our experience of postural yoga. The maturing of our practice can enliven our desire to use the poses (and other means, of course) to establish a relationship with the subtle anatomy and deeper aspects of our mental condition.

Whether we are conscious of it or not, most of us are longing for a direct awareness of our deepest, most peaceful sense of self. The meditative techniques and states of yoga are the "highest," after all. All of our addictions and habits are simply distractions and attachments. They are keeping us from slowing down, reflecting, and inquiring long enough to witness the fruits of the introspective nature of yoga. Our world keeps us engrossed in a fixation on the physical body, and our senses are constantly pulled outward. We are bombarded with sensory input and "food" at all times. However, this physical vessel of the body is a tool to take us inward. We must tend to the vessel to keep it strong and healthy, but from the yogic perspective, we are doing this specifically for our internal development, not for society's external validation.

Naturally, the steps and techniques presented here are moving us from the outer to the inner. The mind likes a systematic approach, and so we can keep the mind somewhat contented as we initially cultivate a healthy physical body and presence in the world through our actions. This creates a fertile foundation for us to begin to clear obstructions of both the physical and mental kind. We can then gently transform ourselves by leaning on the more superior practices by which we uncover the subtle realms of experience. What a delight and a relief even to just *envision* tapping into the seemingly concealed layers of self. Through the process of entrainment, where the techniques each rhythmically fall into synchrony, we begin to slowly unravel our embedded impressions and conditioning. Consider the wealth of freedom that we have access to, if we embark on this dedicated and devotional stairway to the higher and most subtle realms!

Take an opportunity now to consider your personal experience of yoga thus far. How has yoga been presented to you? Taught to you? How has it been represented in marketing or social media? Other than yoga poses, meditation, and "breathwork," what does yoga entail in your eyes? While some are certainly limited, when used in isolation, each of the following components of yoga bears fruits all its own.

Chapter four aims to lay bare the foundational knowledge of varying limbs—beyond Patanjali's renowned eight—that can deepen our acquaintance with yoga. Just as your favorite recipe requires the right ingredients in specific quantities, your personal path will necessitate an individual mixture of techniques and time. This will shift and evolve over months and years. If we zoom out and consider the various stages of life and our unique constitutions, these will ideally guide us to uncover where we need to make adjustments and when.

Just as understanding a historical timeline of yoga (however dry or academic that may seem) can provide a greater frame of reference for the vast field of yoga, embracing a broad spectrum of techniques and practices can also impart an elevated perception. Hopefully it has been made evident that there are many paths and traditions of yoga.

Therefore, know that there is no specific method or strategy you must adhere to. Probably the most beneficial approach to expanding your practice and weaving yoga into daily life is to be consistent. If you do not have the guidance of a skilled teacher, you will be curating your own path to embark on. Repetition and patience will be of great service. The term *abhyasa* may translate to "practice," but at the heart of it, it refers to a *dedicated* practice, one that is receptive and unwavering. It implies that we stay long enough with certain techniques or tools to be able to objectively observe their effects. The mind seeks rapid reward and avoids boredom. Due to this, many of us habitually bounce from one style, teacher, or technique to another. At the other end of the spectrum, some remain attached to a practice that may no longer serve them out of comfort. We must remain in regular reflection and inquiry to access our higher intellect and discrimination.

As you come to understand the following techniques in greater depth, hopefully you will get a strong sense of what you may wish to integrate or *relinquish*. There will be practices that require further instruction from a masterful teacher. This is not intended to be a how-to guide. This information is simply meant to provide further inspiration, to expand your knowledge and potentially set you on a renewed trajectory on your path, one that takes you into the heart of yoga. One that takes you inward.

Sadhana

Sadhana reflects a deeply embedded studentship and dedication. The root *sadh* (SAH-dh) translates to "accomplishing" or "performing." This root word is the basis for the related *sadhaka*. A sadhaka is an aspirant on the path of yoga who has cultivated a way of life and a practice that moves them toward the accomplishment of yoga. It also relates to the Sanskrit word *sadhu* (SAH-du). We often associate *sadhu* with the wandering holy men of India. It is a word that also implies "virtue," "honesty," "benevolence," and "honor." You may therefore get a sense that sadhana requires a genuine commitment to and reverence for the path. To apply oneself to any practice that is rigid and dogmatic will never be sadhana. Sadhana reflects a conscious desire to move in the direction of a spiritual goal. It may be a set of practices or a lifestyle that increases the probability of success and accomplishment.

A sadhana is a practical path that evolves through spiritual maturation to revelation. Certain principles need to be in place for a personal practice to bear reliable results. This is why a generic postural yoga practice does not constitute sadhana. While everyone has the potential to be a sadhaka (a spiritual aspirant engaged in sadhana), of course not everyone has to be. These concepts do not need to convey some kind of exclusivity. However, it is important to refine how we understand these terms so we can use them with greater integrity—and know when to avoid them.

You may have heard or read the saying that suggests making all of your *life* a sadhana. What does this actually mean? It may seem like a lofty goal, as if you would need to renounce the world and all of its pleasures. However, it is really suggesting that we begin to move away from seeing our rigid formal practices as the only yoga we do. Instead, we can strive to live our daily lives in a way that is in service of our sadhana. For example, consider how our actions, conversations, diet, and lifestyle all have the potential to move us toward our spiritual goal. Life will always test us, and yoga is the application of the wisdom that we receive through the formal techniques or practices, wisdom that we can thread into each moment in a day. The time we set aside for our asana practice or morning meditation, for example, is the easiest time to be composed or operate from the higher intellect. But what about the challenges we face each day: how do we show up in those moments with emotional composure, steadiness, or an easeful regulated breath?

Sadhana must be approached lovingly. When we go too hard or too fast with anything, it increases our chances of falling off course. Unless you are an ascetic, any of the more tangible practices you are engaged in do not need to be aggressive or austere. When we move slowly yet consistently, we are often faced with feelings of boredom, resistance, or simply something blocking us. Yoga sadhana is not intended to be comfortable and serene all the time. Quite the opposite. The journey is to witness the shifting momentum of our vasanas, samskaras, and our karmas as they arise. This witnessing and willingness to show up over and over again is a sign of progress. Observing our perceived stagnation or resistance objectively enables an easier and swifter transformation. We must see ourselves as being in relationship with our sadhana. It breathes a life of its own and has the potential to support us far more deeply than most would realize. Our sadhana is where we take refuge from the world.

Sadhana is a part of both our *dinacharya* (daily routine) and *ritucharya* (seasonal routine). Once cultivated, it becomes a part of the framework of day-to-day life. Sadhana, when defined by a set of techniques, is traditionally practiced in solitude. It takes into account the season, the climate, and the phase of the moon. These connections bring us into greater alignment with an inherent cosmic order. Weaving such rhythmic considerations into all facets of our existence aids us in directly comprehending how to make life sadhana, rather than seeing sadhana as a regimen.

Finally, in addition to the concept of the sadhaka, there is another Sanskrit term that has strong relevance to the yogic path here. *Adhikara* relates to our eligibility to receive the deeper teachings. It alludes to our suitability and qualifications—not of the formal kind on paper, however. Adhikara denotes a certain privilege to access the right teachings at the right time. Again, this is not to suggest exclusivity. More accurately, adhikara is in place to safeguard the nectar of yoga. It ensures that the highest teachings are revealed and passed on to those steeped in unwavering studentship. In the modern and affluent world, we are so used to getting what we want when we want it. However, sampradaya holds strong the long-standing approach to passing on any timeless wisdom. Typically, within the cultural context of Indian life, a masterful teacher decides when a student is ready to acquire certain knowledge and experiences. The process is slow. It allows for thorough assimilation and cultivates patience. It teaches grace and humility. This approach to passing on yogic techniques and wisdom serves the student greatly over the long term.

Self-effort and devotion need to be cultivated to be able to embody and hold steady the sacred secrets of yoga. To have the competence to undertake spiritual study, we may need to first face certain karmas. We may also need to appreciate the stage and season of life that we are in. Our experience and embodiment of yoga will evolve and transform over time. When we shift our internal paradigm around how yoga can be integrated into daily life, we can begin to appreciate that there are many ways to deepen our connection to the holistic and comprehensive tapestry of yoga. Being steeped in yoga's vast landscape does not need to cause any overwhelm. Instead, we can hold ourselves in awe, in reverence, and with the deepest respect for the timeless traditions offered at our feet. Having the grace and dedication to tread slowly yet consistently ensures we will open doors to new levels when the most aligned time arrives. Having this highest trust and this type of faith (shraddha) strengthens our pursuit of spiritual success!

Yama and Niyama

The yamas and niyamas have been made famous within the global yoga community due to Patanjali's eight-limbed ashtanga yoga, as per his renowned Yoga Sutras text. Usually narrowly defined as ethical and moral observances, the five yamas and five niyamas are often interpreted as very rigid guidelines. Through the lens of Patanjali's text, they are presented in a way that may initially seem most relevant to those engaged in renunciation. They appear to urge strict restraint throughout all areas of life. It is significant to emphasize that many other mostly Sanskrit texts from India mention yamas and niyamas. For example:

> SATYAM VADA | DHARMAM CHARA ||
> SVADHYAYANMAPRAMADAH ||
>
> *Speak the truth, pursue your inherent duty and never sway from self-study.*[13]

In fact, these observances date far back to the Rigveda. On average, the various texts refer to ten yamas and ten niyamas instead of Patanjali's five of each. In the simplest sense, these ethical and moral principles are the foundation of embedding yoga firmly into our daily lives. We do not have to view them as harsh limitations. We may choose to study them, not only through the traditional perspective, but also through one that complements our present-day world—that is, the perspective of the most common householder tradition.

Yamas and niyamas can guide us into greater mental stability and healthy and harmonious relationships of all kinds, and they can foster a sense of inner peace. Just as young children benefit from boundaries, we can too. Yoga cannot transpire without a degree of ethical and moral conduct. If we cannot—or will not—tend to the quality of our relationship with the external world, any spiritual pursuit can be fueled by false virtue or pretense. Senior teacher Donna Farhi explains it well:

> The yamas and niyamas are emphatic descriptions of what we are when we are connected to our source. Rather than a list of do's and don'ts, they tell us that our fundamental nature is compassionate, generous, honest and peaceful.[14]

The Sanskrit word *yama* translates to "rein," "rule," "curb," "self-restraint," or "observance." Yama is also the god of death, who will permanently rein you in at some point in the future. *Niyama* translates to "restriction," "controlling," "preventing," or "voluntary penance." The highly regarded Mahabharata epic and its substory, the Bhagavad Gita, list many traits and methods of conduct to abide by. Tantrik texts (such as the *Sharada Tilaka*) alongside the influential Hatha Pradipika mention twenty observances in total. The ten mentioned in the Yoga Sutras are merely the tip of the iceberg, so to speak. Nonetheless, the yamas are generally seen as how we interact with others and engage in the world. The niyamas reflect personal and sometimes private observances.

The most common yamas are as follows.

AHIMSA

Normally translated as "nonviolence," this term classically relates to the cardinal virtue in Buddhism and Jainism: not injuring anything. In a broader sense, it can relate to many aspects of how we engage within society. This commonly includes the food we consume—*ahimsa* is a popular term used by those who abide by a vegetarian or vegan diet. A *vegetarian* sattvic diet is the one generally encouraged within most yogic traditions, but absolutely not always. Ahimsa also relates to not intentionally hurting anyone through our words, written or spoken. Unfortunately, the internet can be an ugly realm of appalling communication at any given time, and understandably, no matter how hard we try, we cannot control the emotional conditioning and responses of others. Therefore, the emphasis here is on our genuine intent.

Ahimsa is also associated with how we avoid harm to the earth (and its atmosphere) as best as we can. Importantly, we must not get too aggressive or dogmatic about this, because that can cause self-harm or otherwise build division between ourselves and others who choose to live a different path. The risk with personal interpretations of ahimsa is that it can create a sense of moral superiority. This type of self-righteousness does not help anyone progress along the spiritual path. In addition, to ensure we are not harming ourselves through word and deed is equally valuable in the embodiment of ahimsa. Ahimsa is considered to be the supreme dharma, as is reflected in the phase *ahimsa paramo dharma*, which is attributed to the epic Mahabharata as well as a number of teachers. Thankfully, classical texts also highlight what one is to do when faced with war, the need for self-defense, and determining proportionate punishment within society.

SATYA

Truth and honesty are the most common interpretations of *satya*. It reflects a sincerity behind our words and actions. To embrace satya is to act in alignment with what is virtuous and with the greater cosmic order. It is not only about speaking what is true, although that is important, if done with kindness and integrity. To act consistently in response to the things we say is also an aspect of truth. To deceive or withhold information from another can also be a breach of truth. Satya regulates the universe. The Vedas hold it as necessary to ensure *rta* (the natural harmonious order of nature). We can begin by aligning all of our thoughts, words, and actions with what is factually correct. Emotional neutrality is paramount here. This is simply a means to move toward our inherent true nature and higher Self (Brahman = Sat). *Asat* is the Sanskrit word denoting the opposite: "delusion," "falsehood," or "wrong knowledge." This is beautifully articulated through the following mantra and prayer:

> ASATO MA SADGAMAYA |
> TAMASO MA JYOTIRGAMAYA |
> MRTYORMA'MRTAM GAMAYA ||[15]

This is widely translated as follows:

> *From the unreal lead me to the real,*
> *From the darkness lead me to the light,*
> *From death lead me to immortality.*

ASTEYA

Also called *achaurya*, *asteya* refers to "non-stealing." It implies a virtuous self-restraint that indicates not only abstaining from any kind of theft but also any desire or *intention* of stealing. In today's world, stealing isn't just limited to physical items. It also relates to the theft of another's identity, thoughts, words, work, and even their *time*. Plagiarism is a far-too-common occurrence in our media-driven world. On the path of yoga as we are learning and assimilating knowledge from our teachers, we may at times regurgitate their insight as if it were our own as we attempt to assimilate it. This is natural. However, passing something off as one's own to others is acting outside of integrity. This is why it is also respectful to acknowledge our teachers, lineage, or tradition of teachings. No one owns yoga. However, this is not an excuse to claim ownership over any particular teaching or method. Generosity is regarded as an antidote to asteya, and non-attachment can breed generosity.

In chapter 2 of Patanjali's Yoga Sutras, *Sadhana Pada*, we find the following teaching:

> ASTEYAPRATISHTHAYAM SARVARATNOPASTHANAM || 2.37 ||
>
> *On being firmly established in non-stealing, all kinds of wealth present themselves.*[16]

An alternative word for "wealth" (Sanskrit: *ratna*) would be "jewels" or "gems." It is in the above translation that we come to understand that wealth isn't limited to the material (there are "*all kinds* of wealth"). Furthermore, a greater teaching here reflects that the yogi is offered this wealth—such as food, money, or a place to sleep—as a way that the people of the community, the householders, can show respect and devotion toward the practitioner. Meanwhile, the yogi holds no attachment to anything received.

BRAHMACHARYA

Traditionally translated to suggest a vow of celibacy, the word *brahmacharya* is also used to denote the earliest stage of life in the four ashramas. This vow of celibacy is not merely a lifelong restraint from sexual activity. It also reflects full control of both the body and mind. It is to conquer all desire. It is to conduct oneself in a way that is consistent with Brahman, or the highest state of consciousness. Retention of sexual fluids is believed—in *some* yoga traditions—to assist in cultivating the strength and capacity to attain certain yogic states. Within the context of the yamas, and in our current world, the term most appropriately indicates careful consumption or mindful indulgence in the senses. We must appropriately conserve our energy, our prana, in all thoughts and actions. Rather than full abstinence from sexual activity, we may alternatively operate in a way that is controlled, thoughtful, and respectful of ourselves and others. Through the lens of brahmacharya, any activity (especially sexual) that dissolves our life force deserves foresight and careful consideration. We must always contemplate if our choices will bring us joy or are intended to fill an internal void.

APARIGRAHA

Literally translated to "renouncing" or "deprivation," the Sanskrit *aparigraha* indicates nonpossessiveness. It intends to convey the valuable consideration of keeping what is only sincerely necessary and significant at each stage of life. It also relates to any obsessive possession of or grasping onto people, relationships, and roles. While on first investigation aparigraha usually appears to represent the extremes of asceticism, it has immense value to any householder.

In our current world where it seems we can have it all, aparigraha signals us to employ strong discernment. Giving up greed and the hoarding of physical possessions is a fertile foundation. When we die, we take nothing with us. Yet, the senses keep us strongly attached to our stuff and the identity associated with those things. For the average person, many of the things we own we could easily do without. For some, possessions are a way to cover up internal trauma. Possessions help us avoid confronting the reality of impermanence. Regardless, most of our stuff, beyond the genuine essentials and a few truly meaningful items, gives us a false sense of safety and security, and the pursuit of more drains our life force.

This non-grasping also relates to thoughts and behaviors we cling to as though they were addictions. No doubt we all have emotions and limiting beliefs we could relinquish. The global trend of minimalism is a reflection of the excessive obsession with possessions we are witnessing.

We reclaim more time and mental freedom through owning less. The process of letting go does not have to be extreme. We all need certain things to sustain us at any given time. Taking time for reflection on all we accumulate, acting on that discernment, and leaning on restraint, we can experience the lightness that aparigraha offers.

Some of the additional yamas that are found across Upanishadic, Tantrik, and Hatha texts are the following:

KSHAMA: "Patience" that promotes forgiveness. Tolerance.

DHRTI: "Will," "holding," and "firmness" that inspire perseverance and fortitude.

DAYA: "Compassion" that cultivates a desire to mitigate others' difficulties.

ARJAVA: To be "frank," "straight," "sincere," and transparent with others.

MITAHARA: Regarding intake, this denotes the consumption of a "moderate" amount of food, or a "scanty diet." It suggests satisfaction. It also extends beyond the food we eat and relates to the mental impressions we consume from our environment.

KRPA: "Compassion" and "tenderness."

Note that *shaucha* is sometimes listed as a yama, depending on the text. However, we will address it in the list of niyamas, as it is more commonly known within Patanjali's Yoga Sutras.

The customary niyamas are as follows:

SHAUCHA

Literally translated to "cleanliness" and "purity," *shaucha* (often also written as *sauca* or *saucha*) traditionally indicates a physical purification of the body. Additionally, it implies a clean and clear mind. Daily ablutions are woven into the fabric of the everyday rhythm in India. It is customary to bathe in holy waters near any sacred temple before going inside. This could even be as simple as walking the feet through water at a temple entrance, if there is no large body of water nearby. It is deemed essential to wash before conducting any ritual such as puja or yajna. A light daily cleaning of the home altar is an essential aspect of Indian culture. The discipline that cultivates external and internal purification results in the presence of sattva. Purification may involve not only showering or bathing, but also various techniques found in Hatha yoga and Ayurveda. This could include any combination of tongue scraping, kriyas such as nauli or neti, enemas, yoga postures, pranayama, meditation, and more. *Shuddhi* is a common synonym for *shaucha*.

SANTOSHA

Santosha translates to "satisfaction" or "contentedness." It reflects a state of mind that is unruffled by surroundings, company, or polarities (such as pleasure and pain). You may begin to get a sense of how many of the yamas and niyamas are in relationship with each other. For example, asteya is a foundation for the experience of santosha. Requiring the detachment and dispassion of vairagya, santosha frees us from compulsion. It liberates us from—in modern-day lingo—FOMO (the "fear of missing out"). Santosha frees us from craving, and thereby we begin to be freed from bondage.

When we spend enough time regularly immersed in quietude and introspection, contentedness comes more easily. We are less inclined to run away from our inner struggles or resistance. If we are faced with the projection of someone else's anger or pain, we can do our best to choose composure and see the interaction as an instruction—an opportunity to uncover some kind of lesson or insight. With this resolve, we are more likely to understand the circumstance objectively and remain detached. Simultaneously, we must not use this as a disguise or an excuse to become avoidant.

TAPAS

A word often associated with renunciation or the path of a Hatha yogin, *tapas* is translated as "warmth," "heat," "penance," or "bodily mortification." Also called *tapasya*, this niyama is linked to the burning away of one's karmas through austere practices. It may also relate to the internal fire that is cultivated through the Hatha techniques. In a practical sense for the present-day student of yoga, tapas is pursued through discipline. Realistically, this is of the less comfortable kind. Not that we need to engage in the extreme acts of ascetics. Instead, we are forcing ourselves out of bed to do our practice, or puja, even if we don't feel like it. Maybe we are holding a long-term commitment to a specific daily mantra sadhana. It is a commitment to some kind of discipline that will see us challenged and face resistance, more than once. It is holding the spiritual fruits of the goal in mind and not allowing the mind to be the master. Tapas may involve the ongoing application of a "remedy" that is advised by a *Jyotishi* (Vedic astrologer). It is an act, usually performed in solitude, that will eventually aid us in neutralizing karmas and move us closer toward a spiritual objective.

SVADHYAYA

Often suggested to mean "Self-study" or "Self-inquiry," *svadhyaya* translates to "sacred recitation and repetition of the Veda," "recitation of any sacred text," or "repeating the Veda aloud." It denotes introspection and reflection that is inspired by the direct study of yogic scripture (which is addressed in chapter five). This study of shastra is emphasized as a means to preserving the timeless wisdom of the Veda.

Sva means "one's own" and refers to our essential nature. *Adhyaya* means "lesson," "reading," or "lecture." It is significant to note that svadhyaya is not simply the gathering of Vedic knowledge. It is not about retention of information. The in-depth and ongoing sincere study of Self (via the traditional texts) should guide us in navigating life's difficulties. Svadhyaya should help us experience a feeling of steady assurance. It can eventually bring us into such deep introspection that we unlock the door to higher states. The transmission of knowledge pulls us into a relationship with *Self*—the true nature of reality. So, while a broad definition may indicate inquiring into our traits, karmas, or conditioning, at its core svadhyaya is intended to be the study of sacred texts that awakens a direct perception of the Supreme Reality.

ISHVARAPRANIDHANA

Sometimes written as *Ishvara pranidhana*, this term translates from Sanskrit to "devotion to God." *Ishvara* means "Supreme being," "God," "ruler," or "Lord." *Pranidhana* means "prayer," "access," "applying," and "attention." These quite literal translations can feel far too religious for some, however. More secular interpretations of this niyama tend to suggest acceptance, remembrance of grace, a surrender to the larger order, the offering of the fruits of our efforts to a higher purpose, and a devotion to the fundamental source that connects us all.

If you *are* comfortable with the idea of the personification of a Supreme Reality or higher consciousness, the concept of *ishta devata* is useful. This term refers to the divine form that you feel most connected to. Your ishta devata may be given to you by your guru or passed down through family lineage. But if you were not born in India, neither of these is likely. In which case, through your own studies and circumstances, you may come to feel a strong connection to a particular form of the divine. This might be one that is well-known, such as Ganapati (Ganesha), Shiva, Krishna, Hanuman, or Durga. You may also consult a Vedic astrologer for guidance on discovering the most agreeable ishta devata for you. You may then choose to meditate on or recite a Vedic mantra for your chosen divine form. In doing so, you can bring their most virtuous and wholesome qualities to life within yourself.

Some additional niyamas found across various texts are:

HRI: "Modesty" and humility.

DANA: "Act of giving" or "donation." It reflects charity and sharing with others in need.

MATI: The development of mindful reflection, "intelligence," and "perception" to reconcile and bring "resolution."

ASTIKYA: "Piety," a "faith" and unwavering "belief" in God, guru, spirit, the goal, or higher consciousness.

SIDDHANTA SHRAVANA: A listening to or study of (*shravana*) yogic scripture and "established treatise" (*siddhanta*).

ISHVARAPUJANA: "Worship," "honor," and "reverence" (*pujana*) toward the "Supreme" or "God" (Ishvara). This may also imply the act of ceremonial puja.

VRATA: The firm upholding of a "vow" or "holy practice."

HUTA: Something "offered in fire," or making a "sacrifice" or "offering." This can pertain to the physical acts of Vedic fire rituals like puja, homa, and yajna but could also be an internal oblation.

JAPA: The "muttering" or "whispering" of repetitive mantra recitation.

Generally speaking, the yamas are considered to be ways we should interact with others, or how we uphold ourselves when engaged in contact with another. Niyamas are seen as internal acts to adhere to and therefore regulate the mind. However, what may be equally beneficial (if not of foremost importance) is to direct each of the yamas toward ourselves: for example, to abstain from harmful thoughts or deeds and to be honest with ourselves, to value our time and resources, to stop any depletion of our energy through excess sensory indulgence, or to live simply with freedom from excess and attachments. These are all ways to potentially apply yama to oneself. After all, the Sanskrit words *yama* and *niyama*, literally defined, indicate a similar approach to any act that requires us to restrict or rein something in.

Shatkriya

Made most famous through Hatha yoga, the shatkriyas are physical acts of yogic purification. They exist with the intent to remove impurities and gain control over some involuntary functions. As a result, the vessel that is the human body becomes more prepared and ready to move along the path and practices of yoga. Possibly having Tantrik origins, the shatkriyas are also known as *shatkarma*. In this context, the words *karma* and *kriya* are synonyms, each implying "action." Related to these techniques are those found in the Ayurvedic treatment known as *panchakarma*. *Pancha* means "five." Panchakarma consists of five well-known cleansing procedures utilized in prescribed amounts, depending on the needs of an individual, for rejuvenation and treatment of disease. Similarly, the shatkarmas (*shat* referring to "six") ideally should be performed under guidance and used in a prescriptive manner that takes into account personal needs, climate, time of day, and season.

Said to be "the most encyclopedic of all the root texts of Hatha yoga," the *Gheranda Samhita* teaches a sevenfold path: purification, asana, mudra, pratyahara, pranayama, dhyana, and samadhi. Here, the shatkriyas are the means to the initial step of purification. This can be known through the following verse:

> SHODHANAM DRDHATA CHAIVA STHAIRYAM DHAIRYAM CHA LAGHAVAM
> PRATYAKSHAM CHA NIRLIPTAM CHA GHATASTHAM SAPTASADHANAM || 1.9 ||
>
> Purification, strength, steadiness, calmness, lightness, realization, and abstraction are the seven means of perfecting the body.[17]

NAULI

Considered to be the king of the kriyas, nauli—also called *naulika*—is a churning of the internal organs of the abdomen. With the feet wide, after an exhalation the central muscles of the abdomen (the rectus abdominis) are engaged to rotate in a clockwise and anticlockwise direction. This churning of the abdomen is unlikely to be learned correctly from a book. Instead, it should be practiced under the guidance of a teacher. Performed on an empty stomach, nauli generates internal heat. It feeds and stabilizes the subtle inner fire. To master nauli, one must gain the correct application of the three major bandhas: *jalandhara*, *muladhara*, and mostly *uddiyana*.

NETI

There are two types of neti. The first is the more common and accessible *jala neti*, which uses water to flush the nasal passages. The second is called *sutra neti*. It is traditionally performed by threading a piece of cotton string into one nostril and drawing it out into the mouth. It is then repeated with the other nostril. Jala neti is deemed far safer and more feasible for the average householder. It uses warm, salty water held in a neti "pot," or vessel. Leaning over a sink or outdoors, the head is tilted to one side with the mouth open. The pot spout is placed over the highest nostril, and the water is poured slowly through it. The water should then begin to come out of the lower nostril. After this process continues for roughly 30 to 60 seconds, the excess water in the nose is blown out. The technique is repeated on the other side.

Jala neti does not need to be done every single morning. In fact, in excess it can cause a dryness of the nasal cavities and an overproduction of mucous to compensate. For this reason, sometimes the presence of excess mucous can be an indication to *discontinue* jala neti, which may seem counterintuitive. Jala neti is best used seasonally as a preventative tool to flush out dust and impurities. The Sanskrit word *neti*, in this context, suggests to "carry away."

KAPALABHATI

Often lumped into the category of pranayama, kapalabhati is mostly intended to purify the sinuses. It can also promote the movement of prana and purification of the nadis within the subtle body. Therefore, it is an excellent tool to prepare the physical body for the subtle practice of pranayama. *Kapala* means "skull" or "cranium." *Bhati* means "splendor," "light," and sometimes "shining." The seated technique involves rapid, forced exhalations with subtle, undetectable inhalations. The abdomen is pumped repeatedly. It is not advised for anyone pregnant or who has high blood pressure or heart conditions.

A slow, consistent approach is important to mastery of kapalabhati. Interestingly, there are a small number of scientific studies currently inquiring into the tangible benefits of this technique on cells and the respiratory system. Kapalabhati is an energizing practice done on an empty stomach, best suited to the morning. It helps to clear congestion, stagnation, and kapha from the body. It supports the mind to rest in steady alertness. When learning this kriya, one can initially feel over-stimulated. With proficiency, kapalabhati will have a calming—but not drowsy—impact.

TRATAKA

Trataka is the "fixing of the eye on an object." Sometimes called "candle gazing" because the object is most often a flame. Performed while seated, trataka is to "look" at or apply one's "gaze" to a selected object such as a yantra, the OM symbol, a black dot, the image of a deity, or another point of focus. Promoting a meditative experience, the chosen object is generally placed at eye level. The yogis suggest it is a technique that promotes better eye health and may relieve insomnia. However, trataka is no doubt a practice that calls forth a purification of the mind and senses through the dissipation of distraction. The object of focus naturally impacts the internal fruits acquired through the kriya.

DHAUTI

The Sanskrit word *dhauti* means "washing." This is an advanced kriya, in which a washed and wet strip of cotton cloth is fed into the mouth, swallowed, and then drawn out of the mouth again. The purpose is to cleanse the digestive tract. However, the word *dhauti* is more of a general term that encompasses multiple techniques. The dhauti that uses a long piece of cloth is the most widely known. For example, one of the three classical Hatha texts, the *Gheranda Samhita*, offers several dhauti techniques that use different tools aside from cotton cloth. Some tend to the digestive tract. Others target different parts of the body, such as the teeth or the rectum.

BASTI

A Sanskrit word that most literally translates to "bladder" or "neck of the bladder," *basti* is a cleansing of the colon. This colonic irrigation is usually done with water through a catheter or tube (*jala basti*). A less common—and perhaps even obscure—technique is to draw air up the colon while seated in *pashchimottanasana*. Hatha texts claim the basti kriya wards off diseases of the urinary system, spleen, and more.

Other Hatha texts mention two additional kriyas, with eight noted in total (*ashtakarma*). One is *gajakarni*, which involves the expulsion of the contents of the stomach. Hatha texts describe the details of this technique a little differently. The other kriya is called *chakri*. It is to cleanse the rectum with turmeric root or one's finger. It is claimed to remove piles, among other benefits.

Understandably, the shatkriyas may seem radical. But we have to remember the context for who, when, and how these techniques were (and still are) used. They must be used with caution and under appropriate guidance. Many serve no immediate need for the householder. We can lean on the more approachable ones, such as jala neti, nauli, and trataka. Regardless, any implementation of the kriyas must always come through an informed lens. We must actively take into account what is best for our unique circumstances at various stages of life.

Vyayama

The majority of transnational postural yoga would fall under the umbrella of *vyayama* (vyah-YAH-muh). The Sanskrit word translates literally to "exercise" or "exertion." It refers to any physical movement that moves the body in various ways and that will eventually cause a degree of fatigue. It relates to the development of self-control of the mind over the body. In the simplest sense, it implies exercise for the sake of physical movement and benefit. Through translation, the word can suggest difficulty, to stretch, to extend, and athletic exercise. In India, a Hindi word for the same activity is *kasrat*.

Vyayama warms the body. It serves to build strength and create greater flexibility. It provides all the benefits that science teaches us about any exercise regime, because it is the same thing. When modern yoga classes present postures in an active, continuous, and dynamic way, we are not so much doing asana but vyayama (to be technically correct). This distinction is not intended to imply disapproval. It is to create clarity and thereby integrity in how we represent the yoga tradition. When we are clear on the intent behind a practice or technique, it becomes far more useful.

We will address asana next, and we will explore it in the true sense of the word as well as through the modern application. However, do keep in mind that the way we often engage with asana reflects vyayama more than it does the "meditative seat" used to progress along the yogic path. Within the context of yoga, what we see expressed as vyayama (which may also serve another purpose, such as tending to the subtle anatomy) generally includes surya namaskar and traditional joint movements.

With a touch of humor, some call these joint movements "old school" yoga. They can be found as a key feature of the Pawanmuktasana series from the Satyananda school of yoga. Predating the Satyananda series, these types of movements are applied in the *sukshma vyayama* practice made popular by Dhirendra Brahmachari, a disciple of the Himalayan yogic master Maharishi Kartikeya. This sequence also includes simultaneous strong, dynamic breathing and is intended to work mostly on the subtle body (sukshma sharira). Related are the *sthula vyayama* techniques. There are five of them, and while they also engage in joint movements, they are evidently more dynamic and appear similar to generic exercises. In addition, they place less emphasis on breathing techniques. The sthula vyayama techniques aim to serve the outer physical body (sthula). These specific movements of the joints are also found in the eighteenth-century C.E. Hatha treatise called the *Hathatattvakaumudi*. In this text written by Sundaradeva, the movements are named *charana*. The text lists ten types and alludes to others of lesser importance. Sundaradeva indicates that the ten charanas help to alleviate disease while increasing prana and internal body heat. We are instructed to practice the charanas a minimum of twenty-five times per day for three months. An excerpt from the text:

> Carana is movement of the limbs which is practised on both sides. Chiefly there are ten caranas. According to the adepts, others are jaghanya (of less importance). Ten types of caranas involve head, stomach, hands, pair of the legs, pairs of thighs and knees. Wrist joints, feet, toes and other joints in the body are prominent ones in jaghanya carana. A wise undertakes the practice of carana meditating on Shiva's dancing form. One rotates the head while touching the chest. One touches the heart (chest) in a manner as if not touched.[18]

Additional verses follow that offer further details of the ten major charanas.

Despite the major cities across India that now reflect a more commodified state of yoga (as per the Western world), you can easily witness these simple exercises and movements performed by an average person in the early mornings, somewhere in a local park or perhaps on a riverbank. Physically, vyayama is incredibly valuable for the modern body and lifestyle. Our physical vessel needs movement. This type of exercise supports all systems of the gross body, reduces tamas, and moves prana more sufficiently. Even better is when we utilize it through an Ayurvedic lens. In this case, hopefully it will lead us to a steadier and more comfortable seat—asana—for meditation.

Asana

How did yoga evolve to look as it does in the world today? What are the origins of postural yoga, this "asana"-dominant approach? How did we get here? Hopefully, these considerations were somewhat clarified in chapter one. You would likely agree that the postural-focused yoga practice of today does not really resemble the yoga from which it claims to be derived. Both practitioners and outsiders alike often have little awareness that this transnational modern yoga has no precedent within the Indian yoga traditions. When we see so much of yoga—especially within the online sphere—we often cannot help but think it looks a lot like gymnastics. Given the historical timeline of yoga, this interpretation is likely quite accurate. The posture-heavy approach to yoga has developed and evolved through the influence of both European and Scandinavian gymnastics, bodybuilding, and the YMCA physical culture movement within India itself. Therefore, this approach to yoga is very much a synthesis of both Eastern and Western influence and sits primarily within a Hatha yoga framework. But is it really *asana*?

First, let's inquire into the purpose of yoga postures. The vast majority of people associate the postural practice of yoga with health and wellness, which includes physical flexibility, mobility, strength, stability, and balance. Nowadays, it is also considered to reduce mental stress. If you are more acquainted with yoga studies, you will appropriately associate the postural practice with a reduction of tamas. In addition, through it we experience the mitigation of a busy, distracted, excited, or agitated mind—the mental manifestation of rajas.

Consider that the main purpose of yoga postures, however, especially through a Tantrik lens, is the modulation of prana. In today's chaotic world, perhaps we need not concern ourselves with directing prana into specific parts of the body. Rather, we may simply focus on the maintenance of efficient circulation of prana throughout the entire body. This is where intelligent sequencing of postures (called *krama*) is imperative. This has nothing to do with "peak poses," "funky flows," or a physical goal of sorts. Performing postures in *combination* with bandha, kumbhaka, and mudra can take us toward this key purpose of the postures (that is, pranic modulation).

To modulate prana through postures we must understand the influence of various spinal movements and pose categories. This involves forward folds, lateral sideways movements, backbends, twists, and inversions. Each influences the five vayus that are responsible for all basic bodily functions. You may therefore wonder which postures are most beneficial to integrate into a personal practice and sadhana. In the earliest texts that refer to any postures, we know that seated poses were the first ones practiced. This is generally because a yogic path primarily concerned itself with seated pranayama and meditation. The Sanskrit word *asana* translates to "seat." Also "stopping," "halting," and "dwelling." With that knowledge alone, we can appreciate that the original intent behind asana was likely to cultivate a seat in which to be still and to dwell in meditation. Other than seated poses, the earliest additions to the small list of asanas were some arm balances, inversions, and supine positions. Standing poses were the last to find their way into yoga. Also, the inversions we see in older texts are normally regarded as *mudras*, not asanas. More on that in the forthcoming section on mudras.

In our present-day world, inversions have become far more superficial than ever intended. Certainly, there can be real benefits in the physical challenge of inversions for some yoga practitioners. Even more so in the mental challenge of facing our fears (and doubts around our capacity) when the body is turned upside down. However, at the heart of it, inversions were and are intended to be therapeutic and held for extended durations. The inversions that are generally most revered are *viparita karani*, *sarvangasana* (shoulderstand), and *shirshasana* (headstand). Headstand and shoulderstand are sometimes nicknamed the "king and queen" or the "head and heart" of yoga postures.

To shed light on the Ayurvedic application of yoga postures provides even greater enrichment and benefit. If we imagine that our body is the vehicle that carries us along the path toward the highest state of yoga, Ayurveda is the mechanic that tends to the health and longevity of that vehicle. Inextricably linked, these "sister" disciplines create a holistic approach for our health and spiritual success. When developing or adjusting a personal practice (postural or otherwise), we benefit tremendously from the consideration of the principles taught within Ayurvedic lifestyle practices.

The main considerations are:

TIME OF THE DAY: Each 24-hour cycle is broken up into six parts, each with its own qualities that we can work with.

TIME OF THE YEAR (SEASON): The seasons bring distinct qualities that influence our mental and physical well-being. Hence our practice can balance and harmonize any excesses or depletions when working with seasonal qualities.

WEATHER: Climate can vary from day to day within any season. For example, a sunny day has a distinctly different quality from a rainy one, even within the same season.

PERSONAL CONSTITUTION (PRAKRITI): This reflects our inherent tendencies and needs.

CURRENT STATE (VIKRUTI): This reflects any present imbalance or dominant influence on our state at any given time.

MENSTRUAL CYCLE: The entire menstrual cycle is, like the time of day, broken up into phases dominated by different qualities. We can adapt any practice to support these fluctuations.

EXISTING HEALTH CONDITIONS: We take into consideration any physical or mental health ailments. This includes even mild conditions such as the common cold.

When our movement and exercise choices are applied through a seasonal and constitutional lens, they become Ayurvedic in nature. These considerations also apply to other components of the yoga practice, such as pranayama.

Worthy of attention within any contemplation around asana are karanas. Karanas are widely recognized as the remarkable 108 positions or movement phases seen carved on a handful of ancient South Indian temples. These ornate carvings are perhaps most famously seen at the Chidambaram Nataraj temple in Tamil Nadu, which is a holy pilgrimage site for devotees of Lord Shiva. Also called Thillai Nataraja temple, it is dedicated to Shiva and his form of Nataraj, the Lord of Dance. Carved into the eastern *gopura* wall, Chidambaram temple shows all 108 karanas (other temples may not feature the full number). Interestingly, the temple is regarded as the most subtle of the five elemental *linga* temples. Chidambaram represents the element of akasha—space or ether.

The karanas are described in the esteemed *Natya Shastra* text by Bharat Muni. Often regarded as an additional Veda, it is an ancient and primary treatise for India's performing arts. The 108 karanas are considered to be a means to spiritual freedom or enlightenment. This is in contrast to any other regional, folk, or modern performing arts styles of India. No one really knows exactly how they were performed in ancient times. Many innovations and interpretations have led to the development of codified classical dance forms in India, such as Bharatanatyam and Odissi. Drawing on the *Natya Shastra*, the temple carvings, other texts, and dialogue with the *devadasi*, these dance styles teach what is deemed sacred geometry. They embrace both masculine (*tandava*) and feminine (*lasya*) qualities within the body movements and positions. The devadasi were female artists devoted to and married to the Lord. In service to the deity, they usually resided in temples to perform for the murti (idol) every day while also tending to the care of the temple. This was not a public performance as we know dance and the arts to be conducted today.

The Sanskrit word *karana* literally means "doing," "action," or "causing." In the words of Shandor (Sundernath) Remete, it is regarded as an "instrumental form of transformation."[19] Despite the karanas having been innovated upon in the classical Indian dance styles, in the true sense of the word, the karanas are mostly standing positions where the upper and lower limbs operate in a kind of proportional and synchronistic relationship. Given that we see the karanas portrayed statically on temple walls or in texts, we may be led to believe they are fixed, stationary poses. However, they are coordinated, precise positions in movement. They are actions in a kind of transition. In a sense, they could be likened to the synchronistic movement of surya namaskar or the present-day style of vinyasa. The karanas are classically attributed to Nataraja (Lord Shiva). The prominent pose we see Lord Nataraj in—you likely have seen a statue or image of it in a yoga studio—is the karana called *bhujangatrasita*. Although visual depictions of the karana may not resemble the yoga postures we know today (albeit there are a few that look rather similar), the way they were performed is likely comparable.

The Hatha Pradipika text references karana, kumbhaka, and asana all at once in a key aphorism found within the first chapter:

> PITHANI KUMBHAKASHCHITRA DIVYANI KARANANI CHA |
> SARVANYAPI HATHABHYASE RAJAYOGAPHALAVADHI || 1.67 ||

> The various asanas, kumbhakas and other divine karanas [procedures] of hatha, are to be practiced until the fruit of raja yoga is attained.[20]

Practically speaking, the karanas are an aid to transition us from the standing postures of yoga to the seated. In addition to this, their fundamental purpose of moving us toward spiritual liberation is no doubt parallel to the objective of yoga postures in general. Here are some insightful words from Shandor (Sundernath) Remete, an initiate of the Kanphata Hatha yogins of Nepal and a highly respected teacher globally, that further illuminate the essence of the karana:

> Karanas were used in slow rhythmic movements to gain mastery over the opposing aspects of sthiti (static) and ghati (dynamic) movements which are the basis of all life. Action and inaction are interwoven; motion is resolved in stillness and stillness dissolves into motion. Mastery of the karanas brings the reward of voluntary control over the hitherto involuntary functions of the body. This is a fundamental requirement for beginning the absorption (meditative) practices of yogasana.[21]

To revert back to asana in its truest sense within Patanjali's Yoga Sutras, we are reminded that asana should reflect *sthira* and *sukha*: sthira-sukham asanam || 2.46 ||

Sthira implies "still," "settled," and "calm." *Sukha* suggests "comfort," "ease," and "pleasure." So, if asana is a seated posture for meditation, it is therefore one that should be comfortable and that promotes stillness. In this state, we can relax all efforts. To cease any sense of exertion, only then are we able to dissolve our thoughts and facilitate the subtle practices of yoga. A strained seat only further agitates the mind. Hence, we circle back to the essential value of modern postural yoga as a means to facilitate the physical comfort that allows us to access asana as originally intended. Beyond that, however, the postural practice also holds the potential to develop greater proprioception, interoception, and spatial awareness, which aids in optimum physical functionality and longevity in daily life.

Mudra

Mudra is often simplified to reflect simple hand or finger gestures. These *hasta* mudras have origins in Indian dance, as per the *Natya Shastra*. They usually denote deep symbolism. Hand gestures are used extensively in classical dance and drama in India for aesthetics and storytelling as well as symbolism. Therefore, they should never be appropriated into another performing art form without a nuanced understanding prior (at the least). Hasta mudras are also commonly used in meditation, nyasa, pranayama, pratyahara, and puja. Each finger represents one of the five elements and is considered to emanate rays of our solar energy. Each finger also represents a *graha* (planet), as per Vedic astrology and hasta samudrika.

In reality, the subject of mudra is extensive and diverse. Mudras are much more than hand gestures. They can be expressed through the face, mouth, tongue, and the entire body—this even includes the anus. Even bandhas are regarded as mudras. The word *mudra* is most commonly believed to be of Sanskrit origin, composed of *mud* and *dra* or *dru*. Alternatively, it has been argued that the word may have Tamil or Dravidian roots. Regardless, the Sanskrit word *mudra* translates to "seal," "stamp," "impression," or an "image" or "sign" (in the case of a mark of divine attributes being placed on the body).

Mudras are used to focus and direct our awareness. They are engaged to bind, direct, and redirect prana within the subtle body. This energy is then attentively held in a specific location for an extended duration. As a result, prana—and power—is intensified. This process has a direct influence on our capacity to arouse kundalini. Mudras help to remove obstructions of the subtle body so that it is further strengthened. Knowing this, you may appreciate the value in mudras of the entire body, not only the hands. In fact, across Hatha texts, gestures of the hands are rarely emphasized.

It is significant to highlight that this section on mudras (and the subsequent section on bandhas) would be more correctly positioned *after* pranayama. Bodily mudras are a bridge between the physical and subtle, or the outer and inner, practices. Outwardly, mudras and bandhas appear more physical and tangible; therefore, their discussions are placed between those of asana and pranayama in this book. However, at the heart of it, they could be said to belong after pranayama. It is through the use of asana or karana *with* varied pranayama techniques that we effectively create mudra. A mudra stimulates a process by which the subtle body is refined and pranic obstructions are eradicated. Please keep this in mind as you proceed and assimilate the subsequent guidance.

Familiar mudras that you may have already used include the placement of the tongue in *shitali* (shee-ta-lee) pranayama or the hand placement in *shanmukhi* mudra. Perhaps the most common would be *namaskara* and *anjali* mudras, placing the hands in a prayer position. Some of the most important mudras for a yoga practitioner are as follows:

MAHAMUDRA: A seated mudra that engages the three major bandhas (which we will expand on in the following section), mahamudra is used to liberate pranic blockages in the lower chakra centers. It frees us from thoughts and behaviors of the lower mind associated with the consumption of food, alcohol, and sex, for example. The three bandhas involved are jalandhara, uddiyana, and mulabandha. These bandhas are also engaged in unison in mahabandha. The simplest difference between mahamudra and mahabandha is the position of the seat. Mahamudra is performed seated with one leg extended in front. The other is bent, with the foot placed on the inner upper thigh and the knee externally rotated. The hands clasp the foot of the straight leg. The spine is erect, despite a slight forward fold. Certain breath patterns are engaged, and the three bandhas are applied depending on the stage of breath (or retention).

VIPARITA KARANI: The Sanskrit word *viparita* means "inverted" or "reversed." Therefore, all inverted postures can be—and sometimes traditionally are—called *viparita karani*. Especially shirshasana (headstand). Note that the *karani* here can be linked back to *karana*, as per the previous section on asana. Predominantly, viparita karani is a mudra performed lying down with the legs extended up in the air, slightly bent, and the hands supporting the pelvis. From the side, the pose creates a broken line (rather than a straight line, as in headstand or shoulderstand). It is a full-body mudra, rather than an asana (or the like). It is an active pose that, over time, promotes equilibrium. Due to its inverted nature, the mudra supports the movement of prana into and up the central channel. This potentially includes the reversal of apana vayu (when intended). The mudra promotes a reabsorption through the reversal. Generally, this is the reabsorption or retention of the amrita, or nectar, found in the head. Viparita karani promotes sensory withdrawal and thereby has a calming impact on the mind.

KECHARI MUDRA: This is an advanced mudra essential to learn under the guidance of a teacher. It is especially prized within Hatha yoga. Kechari curls the tip of the tongue up to the soft palate and back toward the nasal cavity. A short frenulum, otherwise known as a tongue tie, can restrict access to the mudra. Yogis used to intentionally stretch, "milk," and massage their tongues. They would eventually severe the frenulum if deemed necessary. The main purposes of the mudra are to control the movement of prana and to access amrita in the head. Kechari is considered to be the "king" of mudras, though it is sometimes called the "queen" to reference its more feminine quality and relationship to kundalini. Kechari is of supreme importance, as it is likened to a switch between the physical and subtle.

Other mudras you may uncover through texts or practice could be those such as *ashwini*, *kaki*, *maha vedha*, *shambhavi*, or perhaps *shakti chalana*. If you ever sit to observe yagna or puja in a temple, you may witness multiple hand mudras gestured throughout by the *pujari*—the temple priest whose duty is to perform puja.

Bandha

As mentioned previously, the three major bandhas are internal mudras. In combination, they give rise to mahabandha. The bandhas can serve to free the granthis, move stagnant prana, direct and hold prana, or otherwise control kundalini. The Sanskrit word *bandha* translates to "binding," "contracting," "a bond," "capture," and to "tie." These bandhas were likely developed through Tantra and out of the desire to work with an inner alchemy. More than mere physical contractions, they tend to the metaphysical system of the vayus (winds), as discussed in chapter two. In their most advanced stages, the bandhas awaken dormant spiritual energy within. Harnessed during breath retentions, they work like taps or safety valves.

MULABANDHA: *Mula* means "root" and "foundation." Mulabandha is a contraction of the pelvic floor, generally speaking. It is described with slight differences depending on the text. Nonetheless, the bandha is ultimately intended to force apana vayu back upward toward the abdomen to fan the inner subtle fire. This is in an effort to reach prana vayu and eventually ignite the active state of kundalini. Usually performed seated during a breath retention after exhalation, mulabandha can be utilized to some degree while in movement and also during a breath retention after inhalation.

JALANDHARA BANDHA: Commonly called a chin lock, jalandhara bandha is engaged when the chin is contracted and drawn downward to the base of the throat. The chin tucks toward the uppermost chest area to lock or redirect prana. *Jala* means "net," among many other things. This likely conveys that jalandhara is the *adhara* (site) where the net (i.e., the bandha) catches prana. According to Hatha yoga, jalandhara serves to remove blockages of the throat center and helps to control the nadis that extend through the throat and up into the brain. Similar to mulabandha but working in the opposite direction, jalandhara helps to force prana vayu downward into the inner orb of fire. It is normally engaged during a breath retention, after either inhalation or exhalation.

UDDIYANABANDHA: This is the abdominal lock, always performed after exhalation and on an empty stomach. Contraindicated during pregnancy and menstruation, the bandha entails an expansion of the rib cage with a contraction of the belly. The abdomen is vacuumed up, drawing all the organs with it, when executed correctly. The Sanskrit word *uddiyana* means "flying up" or "soaring." During the bandha, the diaphragm is drawn high up into the thoracic cavity. Uddiyana is responsible for the union of prana and apana (due to the union of the previous two bandhas when practiced synchronously).

MAHABANDHA: This bandha is the culmination of proficiency at the previous three bandhas. Performed seated, usually in *siddhasana*, this "great seal" holds all three bandhas together at once after an exhalation. It is said to reduce and clear subtle blockages, namely within the heart and throat centers. It prepares us for the effective practice of mahamudra and mahavedha.

Each of these three bandhas, in isolation and also performed together as in mahabandha, are often regarded as the most important mudras. Their very specific application directly pertains to the breath. This is why, again, the study and practice of mudra and bandha should sit after pranayama and not be perceived as mere physical actions or positions (as they are too often in mainstream yoga).

Pranayama

Through pranayama, we are refining the subtle body and the efficiency of pranic circulation. Still one of the outer limbs of yoga, pranayama grants us closer access to the inner state of dharana (concentration) and beyond. The Sanskrit term *pranayama* comes from *prana* and *ayama*. In this context, *prana* most literally translates to "air," "wind," "respiration," "vitality," or "spirit." It refers to our life force and the subtle energy within every living being. *Ayama* can translate to "stretch," "expand," "lengthen," "restrain," or "stop." Evidently, pranayama is a multilayered term. It would be fair to claim that pranayama intends to convey the extension or expansion of the life force, or that it is a restraint of the breath or the termination of breath without strain (as in *kevala kumbhaka*). Some traditionalists would likely state that any breath technique is not true pranayama until there is integration of kumbhaka on some level. In which case, this could be taken further to say that pranayama is a *state of being*—one that is reflected in a spontaneous cessation of the breath without death. This idea is expressed within Patanjali's Yoga Sutras:

> TASMINSATI SHVASAPRASHVASAYORGATIVICCHEDAH PRANAYAMAH || 2.49 ||
>
> On this (perfection of posture), the cessation of movement of inspiration and expiration of breath is called regulation of breath (pranayama).[22]

This state of effortless breathlessness without death may well be the most supreme control or restraint of the life force. Therefore, within the context of pranayama, prana refers less to the actual physical breath itself, and more to the subtle energy that exists within until we die. Until we get to our moment of death, pranayama ultimately extends and *conserves* our subtle life force. It encompasses a collection of breath techniques, exercises, and patterns that directly impact the subtle body and quality of mind. Even verbal mantra is sometimes considered pranayama, as it can assist in the development of the exhalation and of overall breath regulation (similar to singing). Pranayama aims to purify the nadis (*nadí shuddhi*).

Traditionally, the practice of pranayama came with a strong caution. To manipulate and attempt to restrain the breath can come with significant risks. Therefore, pranayama has—in most cases—been adapted to suit the average householder. Daily integration of pranayama should take into account where the breath is being directed, how long the technique is applied, and how many cycles or repetitions are engaged. Pranayama can stimulate both the sympathetic and parasympathetic nervous systems. Due to this, we need to have a clear understanding of the impact of any technique and what is appropriate at any given time. This includes health conditions, personal constitution, time of day, and the like.

Putting the principle purpose of pranayama aside for the moment, regulation of the breath can have tremendous health benefits for anyone. Our main organ of breath is the lungs. The lungs are our connection to the atmosphere. They are the organ that extracts the essential mix of gases that we require to exist. Lungs are also the frontline of our immune system. This is one extremely valid reason to invest time in the development of effective breathing. After all, lung cancer—which is caused not only by smoking or secondhand smoke—is one of the most common forms of cancer. It kills more people than breast, pancreatic, prostate, and colon cancer combined.

There are 50 million alveoli in the lungs. If you were to take the lung tissue and spread it out, you would be looking at more than 1,500 miles. Yet, wildly, it all fits tucked inside the thoracic cavity. The lungs are the last organ of the body to be developed while we are in the womb, and they do not really kick into gear and fully expand until we take our first breath. Significantly, this breath marks our formal arrival into the world. In contrast, our last breath reflects our final moment of life. However, unfortunately, most of us take our breath for granted and rarely tend to its quality. The breath is a gateway to the brain, thanks to the olfactory system. When we breathe through the nose, we impact our limbic center, which is responsible for our emotional experience. Therefore, when we regulate the breath through the nose, we are also able to regulate our emotional state.

Once the physical body is prepared and comfortable to sit, pranayama can be an effective tool for us to move closer to mental stillness and equanimity. An upright and easeful seated posture enables us to freely access the thin, dome-shaped diaphragm. This sheet of skeletal muscle separates the thoracic cavity from the abdomen. The diaphragm's ability to move well is of utmost importance. We also need the upper chest cavity to have a degree of freedom so we can access the upper lobes of the lungs effectively. The previous shatkriyas evidently help to ready the inner organs and systems. The "asana" and physical movement of yoga allow us to experience greater comfort in being seated with a preferable spinal posture.

Before approaching any pranayama technique or pattern, it is important to understand the four phases of respiration. These are as follows:

PURAKA: References the inhalation and translates to "filling," "completing," "satisfying," and "fulfilling."

ANTARA KUMBHAKA: The breath retention after inhalation. *Antara* translates to "inside," "within," and "in the middle." *Kumbhaka* translates to "pot," which is no doubt an indication of the breath being held or contained (as a pot would hold a substance). The breath is held at the heart or navel center.

RECHAKA: References the exhalation and translates to "emptying," "exhalation," "emitting," and "purging."

BAHYA KUMBHAKA: The breath retention after exhalation. *Bahya* translates to "fear," "dread," and "apprehension." These are all feelings that can arise (and need to be mastered) during an extended pause after dispelling all air from the lungs. The empty breath is "held" at the crown of the head.

It is said that the yogis believe if we have trepidation toward *antara* kumbhaka, we fear our own power. If we feel the same way toward *bahya* kumbhaka, we fear death (i.e., of our conditioned attachment to our identity, possessions, and worldly form).

These four components of pranayama can be applied with varied ratios, even and uneven. *Samavrtti* is the name for even ratios. *Vishamavrtti* ("irregular") refers to uneven ratios. When the breath is entirely suspended without strain, this is the state of *kevala kumbhaka.* Held to be the most superior form of pranayama, kevala (meaning "alone") kumbhaka is when both the inhalation and exhalation are suspended at will. In a sense, it reflects the fundamental purpose of Hatha yoga—the unification of two seemingly opposing forces.

Three noteworthy methods to conduct pranayama are through *anuloma* ("with the grain or hair," suggesting in a natural direction), *viloma* ("against the grain or hair," "inverted," "backward," or "opposed"), and *pratiloma* (also translated as "against the grain or hair," but regarded as a combination of anuloma and viloma, depending on the technique applied). These modes can involve the use of single-nostril breathing, simultaneous nostril breathing, and pauses throughout inhalation or exhalation, and at times the use of a hand mudra (in the case of single-nostril breathing).

Numerous pranayama techniques are listed across yogic texts. Some serve a more physical and therapeutic purpose. Others aim to regulate the mind and its afflictions. Those most consistently given central importance are:

SURYA BHEDANA: In Hatha texts, this technique of "piercing the sun" is the first to be mastered so the other pranayamas can bear their fruits. Surya bhedana places emphasis on inhalation through the right (solar) nostril and antara kumbhaka.

UJJAYI: Translated to "victorious uprising," this well-known warming technique initially requires a gentle internal constriction at the base of the throat, with the mouth held closed. When breathing, the constriction should induce a soft but audible "hissing" sound during *both* inhalation and exhalation. Far too often this technique is aggressively engaged. The result is almost a grunting noise, certainly an excessive sound on exhalation, with hardly any sound during inhalation. This imbalanced and overextended approach is a useless, if not dangerous, application of ujjayi. With mastery, over time ujjayi becomes something far more subtle and further internalized. Victory over respiration is not attained through a strained, loud breath.

NADI SHODHANA: As the name suggests, this technique is the superior way to purify the nadis. *Shodhana* translates to "purifying," "cleaning," "improving," "refining," and "cleansing." It is a word often used in Ayurvedic literature. Known as alternate nostril breathing, the technique uses a right-handed mudra—usually called vishnu or mrigi mudra—to alternatively block the nostrils at the edge of the septum. The right thumb is placed on the right nostril. The ring and little fingers control the left nostril. The placement is associated with the *phana* ("the hood") marma site. Nadi shodhana is similar to—but not the same as—*anuloma viloma pranayama*, despite the names being mistakenly interchanged on occasion.

SHITALI AND SITKARI: These two techniques promote coolness of mind and body. *Shitali* is performed with the mouth open and lips pursed, as in kaki mudra. If possible, the tongue is then slightly poked outward and the lateral edges rolled up together (making a U shape). The inhalation is drawn in through the tongue, then the exhalation is performed through the nose. *Sitkari* is performed similarly. Instead of a rolled tongue, however, the mouth is open with the upper and lower teeth closed and together—much like a fake smile! The hissing inhalation is drawn through the teeth into the mouth. Then the mouth is closed for a nasal exhalation. Yogis claim that sitkari has the added benefit of the elimination of any blood toxicity.

BHRAMARI: "Like a bee," involves blocking the ears by applying *suchi* mudra with the index fingers inside the ears. Or bhramari could integrate shanmukhi mudra, with the thumbs closing off the ears. Either way, the main technique—as there are variations—involves nasal breathing and audible humming on the exhalation with eyes closed. This extended hum develops the breath in a similar way to the verbal recitation of mantra. Bhramari is suggested to facilitate the production of nitric oxide. It eases restlessness and calms the mind. The humming sound pierces our awareness, like a needle, to draw the mind and senses inward.

BHASTRIKA: Like kapalabhati, this technique is easily defined as a kriya also. It helps to remove excess phlegm (kapha) from the entire body, particularly the lungs. It requires a rapid and forceful application of the inhalation and exhalation—similar to an act of hyperventilation but without the anxiety. Although slightly different in technique, kapalabhati could be deemed a gentler or preliminary practice before mastering bhastrika. In Sanskrit, *bhastrika* translates to "bag" or "bellows." The abdomen is rapidly pumped like a blacksmith's bellows. Due to the intense nature of the technique, the breath becomes notably audible (but not aggressive). In some lineages, bhastrika may also be taught with synchronized actions of the arms.

Pranayama is mentioned, and revered, within esteemed yoga shastras such as Patanjali's Yoga Sutras, the Bhagavad Gita, and multiple Hatha and Tantrik texts. You may now have a strong sense that pranayama is akin to a bridge between the more physical techniques and the subtle practices of yoga. Some methods directly serve the gross body; others begin to cultivate the stillness and introspection of the latter limbs.

Pratyahara

Commonly known as "sensory withdrawal," *pratyahara* translates to "retreat," "dissolution of the world," and yes, "withdrawal." According to Patanjali, it is the final stage of the outer limbs, or *bahiranga sadhana*. Pratyahara asks us to gather our awareness and turn it inward, away from distractions that lure the senses. This is to prepare the mind for the subsequent stage of concentration. To control the senses necessitates a degree of mastery of prana. Pratyahara comes from the roots *prati*, meaning "to withdraw," and *ahara*, meaning "food." Hence, we are aiming to reduce the impressions we feed ourselves. In turn, this reduces the mental disturbances we experience. Therefore, perhaps we could label anything that does just this as pratyahara.

Due to this, pratyahara may seem a little mysterious and intangible. If *ahara* refers to all that we take in through the five senses, the practical ways we can apply this withdrawal could be to watch less television, consume less social media, talk and socialize less, eat less, and schedule less. But as they pertain to the yogic path, these acts would be comparable to yamas and niyamas.

In terms of yoga practice specifically, the most known technique of pratyahara is through shanmukhi mudra. This is a beautiful Hasta mudra to symbolically and literally seal the senses. Other practices that could fall into the category of pratyahara are shavasana, yoga nidra, japa (we will address japa in the next section on mantra), Tibetan palming (rubbing the palms to create warmth, then placing cupped hands over the eyes), and *kayaviveka* (physical solitude).

Placed at the end of a postural yoga practice, and occasionally woven throughout (as per Sivananda yoga sequences), shavasana is normally classified as an asana. The pose has the body lying entirely supine on the floor, resting with the eyes closed, and keeping still for several minutes. The posture promotes quietude, stillness, and assimilation of any previous activity. It is often a point of transition between yoga postures to seated pranayama or meditation. *Shavasana* is a Sanskrit word that breaks down into *shava* (corpse) and *asana* (seat). Shava as a corpse is not referring to a literal death of the material body necessarily. Instead, it conjures up a death of the mundane mind—the individual sense of self—and our association with the physical body. The purpose of shavasana is not to take relaxation. Certainly, it is not used as a means to collapse in a postural-yoga-induced heap of exhaustion. After our time in shavasana is complete, we roll to the right intentionally to open the left nostril—associated with the lunar nadi—to further access a state of calm composure.

Yoga nidra is often given the oversimplified title "yogic sleep." It is a technique that aims to uncover the various realms of consciousness. Professed to induce a deep state of mental tranquility, yoga nidra is a process by which we can begin to resolve and dissolve our samskaras. It is a highly accessible yet advanced technique that goes beyond deep relaxation. Only at its initial stage is it pratyahara. It relates to the four states of consciousness and has ties to teachings within the *Mandukya Upanishad*. On the surface, this technique of divine sleep is performed by lying down in complete stillness with the eyes closed. Guided instruction brings one's attention to various sacred sites within the body, and various visualizations offered and adhered to. The practice can begin with a *sankalpa*. *Sankalpa* is usually defined as an "intention," but this resolve is a little more refined and mystical at its heart. Yoga nidra is ultimately a state of being, more so than a technique. It is also regarded as being a goddess, as per the venerated *Devi Mahatmya* text. In fact, yoga nidra is mentioned across much of the revered shastras, such as the Mahabharata and within the more modern *Yoga Taravali*. Through the guided practices that promote pratyahara, we can only then shift into the more subtle states of consciousness—likened to meditation—that take us to yoga nidra.

Kayaviveka is defined as "seclusion" and indicates a physical isolation of the body. For the householder, this would relate to the latter stage of life, when we are encouraged to withdraw from worldly duties. It indicates a retreat from social engagements, conversations, media, and sensory impressions, even if for only short periods each year or perhaps once a month, if feasible.

Pratyahara is not always a clearly defined set of techniques or practices. But when we appreciate the intent and essence, this clarity can reveal the yogic methods that invite us into a genuinely introspective experience. In turn, the subtler realms and embedded conditioning of the mind are eventually illuminated.

Mantra

Within the various Indic traditions, the Sanskrit word *mantra* translates to "instrument of the mind." As transport for *manas* (the mind), *tra* indicates a "tool" or "instrument" of thought. We see this root *tra* also within *tantra* and *yantra*, for example. Mantras are specifically written in the Sanskrit language. Through recitation and correct pronunciation, prana is infused into any mantra. Mantras are not affirmations, and affirmations are *not* mantras. In the Sanskrit language, the meaning of the word *mantra* is described as *mananaat trayate iti mantrah*. This speaks to a sustained repetition of that (the mantra), which protects or transforms.

The only way to keep mantras alive is if we continue to use them. Over time and with ongoing repetition, they have the potential to alter the fabric of space within the body. In addition, mantra helps us to develop and *enjoy* the state of concentration. Hence why this section on mantra sits between pratyahara and dharana. Mantra could therefore fit into either of those categories, depending on our level of established mantra practice.

Vedic chanting is a general term used to refer to the recitation of any text of Indian origin that follows and abides by the integrity of the Veda. These texts fall under the category of smriti, or composed texts—as opposed to *shruti*, the divinely revealed texts (the Vedas). These texts regard the Vedas as the authority. In the context of Vedic chanting, everything is recited according to the language of Vedic Sanskrit. Vedic chanting includes recitation of revered texts such as the Bhagavad Gita and the Yoga Sutras. The inclusion of intonation can vary on a case-by-case basis, owing to lineage or the guided tradition of a primary teacher. As an example, a simple invocation can sound ethereally different between teachers who particularly adhere to the technique of their spiritual lineage.

The most notable difference between Vedic chanting and *Veda* chanting is the fixed intonation. In the Veda specifically, the Sanskrit is marked with the *swara*, indicating the correct note to pronounce. In general, in *Vedic* chanting of other texts, there is no swara or fixed intonation. Intonation in Vedic chanting is generally influenced or directed by the meter. However, the other rules of Veda chanting are to be followed. This is why texts like the Yoga Sutras or the *Devi Mahatmya* may sound different when chanted by teachers of various lineages.

The Veda chanting rules are as follows:

VARNA: Correct pronunciation of syllables.

SVARA: Correct intonation.

MATRA: Duration.

BALAM: Appropriate force.

SAMA: Evenness and continuity.

SANTANAH: Conjunction.

Another variation again is to sing the Vedic mantras, which is not done when reciting any part of the Vedas. When sung or in musical form, Vedic mantras cease to be regarded as "Vedic" chanting. Furthermore, *Veda* chanting is certainly not meant for the purpose of singing. It is virtually impossible to maintain any of the chanting guidelines, and to sing them would dissolve the integrity of the Vedic mantra.

In Veda chanting, one needs to learn from a scholar via direct training with a teacher—one who has been initiated into a Veda *vidyalaya*, a school of Veda. This is to receive specific feedback and correct errors that pertain to the specific guidelines for Veda recitation laid out in the Vedic-era *Pratishakhya* manuals. Here, tradition and lineage are of utmost importance. However, it is not wrong or detrimental to sing certain mantras, such as in the case of devotional bhajans (beautiful songs in praise of God) or kirtan.

While it can be performed solo, kirtan is normally conducted in a group setting, call and response style. It is a practice anchored in Bhakti yoga. The word *kirtana* refers to glorifying the name of the divine. Literally, it translates to "repeating" or "mentioning." Genuine kirtan always involves devotional singing toward a chosen deity, a food offering to the deity, and a distribution of the prasad (blessed food) to participants. Kirtan does not use Veda mantras. Generally, very simple mantras to the deity are sung, such as the often-recognized hare krishna mantra from the *Kali Santarana Upanishad*. Hence, a third type of chanting is called *nitya prarthana*, and refers to general daily prayer, various shlokas, and the like. Perhaps it could be said to be the most informal of the types of chanting.

Aside from the rules and guidelines that pertain to Vedic and Veda recitation, some other guidelines can provide a greater framework and success when chanting. These could include the adoption of a vegetarian diet, which is said to promote lightness and sharpness of mind. Also, mantra recitation is often avoided during the first few days of menstruation to assist in the movement of apana vayu. It is a time to conserve energy and rest.

Many desire the opportunity to receive a personal mantra from a teacher or guru. Typically, this act often pertains to Tantrik traditions (but it can absolutely be a part of others). Of course, it is desirable (although not essential) to be given a mantra from a personal guru. In this case, the mantra is deemed to be infused with shakti (shaktipat). Therefore, an intellectual understanding of the mantra is not considered necessary.

There are various stages of mantra recitation:

VAIKHARI: Repeating the mantra aloud.

LIKHITA: Writing the mantra, while simultaneously reciting it mentally.

UPAMSHU: Whispering the mantra so softly it is inaudible.

MANASIKA: Repeating the mantra inwardly or mentally.

AJAPA: When the mantra (or any sound) arises internally and pulsates spontaneously without effort.

Japa is a technique of repeated mantra recitation or rumination through any of these stages. From the root *jap*, the Sanskrit word means "whispering" or "muttering." These translations allude to the instruction that the mantra should be uttered in a very low, quiet voice. The development of japa recitation can be applied through the stages. The practice may or may not use physical *mala* as an aid. *Mala* (pronounced MAH-lah with *long* "a" sounds) translates to "wreath" or "garland." This should not be confused with *mala* (with short, quick "a" sounds), the Sanskrit word often used in Ayurveda that refers to stool or a bodily excretion.

A *japamala* is usually a looped thread of beads, like a rosary. It has 108 beads or a division thereof, and is made from materials such as wood, gemstones such as clear quartz, stones, or the most prominent, *rudraksha*. Rudraksha is a holy seed, most often worn by Shiva (*Rudra*) devotees. The word *aksha* means "eye." These rudraksha seeds or stones have a varied number of facets, or "faces," called *mukhi*. Whatever the material, note that japamalas are not jewelry. A japamala that is used specifically for mantra recitation is normally worn inside and underneath clothing, with the tassel (or equivalent) worn to the back. It is otherwise held inside a purpose-built bag of sorts. It is deemed personal, sacred, and a tool for sadhana. A garland of beads worn for the purpose of fashion can naturally be worn any way but must not be used for japa recitation.

The technique of japamala involves using the right hand to hold the beaded garland between the thumb and middle finger. The index finger is never used and points away. The place to begin is with the first bead after the main, "guru" bead (where a tassel may attach). The guru bead is down past the thumb. Each bead is held—and sometimes gently rolled or massaged—with each recitation of the mantra. The thumb is the dominant finger that shifts each bead downward with every repetition. A minimum of 108 rounds is performed. If going beyond 108, the beaded garland is flipped around to ensure there is never any chanting on or passing over of the guru bead.

Informally, the word *mantra* is used to describe almost any type of chanting, even the non-Sanskrit kind, such as affirmations and slogans. Unfortunately, this dilutes the essence of mantra. To embrace mantra in its truest sense gifts us with a favorable opportunity to harness the mind more deeply. As we will explore in chapter five, Sanskrit syllables and the entire language at large are regarded as profoundly powerful for altering our internal state. The meaning of a Sanskrit mantra will be internalized over time. It can be an instrument of internal or external worship. It can help us become more acquainted with a deity or sacred shastra. Mantra is a tool to bring us closer to divinity. With sustained, repeated application, a mantra becomes deeply internalized and spontaneous, as indicated by these words from the Indian saint Anandamayi Ma (1896–1982): "Silent Japa should be engaged in at all times. One must not waste breath uselessly: whenever one has nothing special to do one should silently practice Japa in rhythm with one's breathing in fact this exercise should go on continually until doing japa has become as natural as breathing."

Dharana

Dharana is defined upfront in chapter 3 (*Vibhuti Pada*) of Patanjali's Yoga Sutras:

> DESHABANDHASHCHITTASYA DHARANA || 3.1 ||
>
> *Concentration is fixing the mind to one place.*[23]

Contrary to what the mind may perceive, dharana is not something that can be practiced as such. Dharana is a state to cultivate and allow to arise. While certain techniques and objects may aid easier access to dharana, we cannot force the state of concentration to occur. We can only create an environment suited to its emergence. *Dharana* comes from the Sanskrit roots *dha*, meaning to "maintain" or "hold, and *ana*, which translates to "something else." Therefore, dharana refers to the capacity to maintain steady concentration on an object. This relates to *ekagrata*, a term that describes the "intentness in the pursuit of one object" or "close and undisturbed attention." Ekagrata is a single-pointed focus on one thing. You could say then that effective dharana achieves and *maintains* the state of ekagrata.

Dharana refers to the ability to hold concentration on something, but not the object itself. It assists us in witnessing our quality of mind. It is the first stage of *samyama*—the combined, simultaneous experience of dharana, dhyana, and samadhi. In reality, when most people are engaged in a meditation practice, they are likely working at the stage of dharana. Dharana could be considered to be a prelude to meditation in its truest sense, to the state of dhyana. The device used for dharana can be an internal or an external one. Some examples of objects used to develop dharana could be a yantra, a mandala, an image or murti of a deity, the rising or setting sun, the visual OM symbol, the breath—its movement or sound—a short mantra, an awareness of light at a certain location within the body, the sound of bells, a flame in the spiritual heart, and more.

Through developing our capacity to disengage from the outside world (i.e., pratyahara) and find delight with our inner quietude, we can then adhere to an internal focus. This is dharana. If an external object is initially used, over time this advances to holding the image of that same object through our inner eye of awareness. We can see it behind closed eyes. This process requires a letting go. The mind likes to fix itself on rigid techniques or steps, but each practice on the path becomes more subtle and tames the mind to allow for this softening.

Our thoughts, like waves in the ocean, may be present. However, we do not feed them nor need to control them (which is a typical left-brained approach). Instead, the higher mind continues to return to the object of contemplation and concentration. Prana follows wherever the mind goes. This is a stage of the maturation of our yoga practice when we need to release the desire to intellectualize. Instead, we bear witness to and fully embrace the subtle vibratory qualities of existence. We are then able to access the inner light and sound that unfolds through dynamic stillness. "Dynamic" suggests that a lot is happening within the *subtle* realms while we are seemingly physically and mentally still.

At an initial level of establishing dharana, we could use any of the following practices that expand on some of the previously mentioned techniques:

ANAPANASATI: A Buddhist approach—the unbroken observation of breath.

MANTRA JAPA: Repeated recitation of a mantra (as per the previous section on mantra).

TRATAKA KRIYA: Gazing at the tip of a candle flame at eye level. (Revert to the earlier section on the shatkriyas for elaboration.)

PRANA DHARANA: A visualization and directing of prana with light, color, or sensation to establish a concentration of prana at a specific site within the body.

Developing a continual thread of concentration is the first step to the unfoldment of meditation, where the object eventually dissolves. The technique is the tool, but not the state. This is an invaluable discernment to return to. At this stage of yoga, if we have been appropriately dedicated to the earlier facets of the path, this effort (abhyasa) will culminate in dharana. The state of dharana will arise due to the accessible quietening—not necessarily the *removal*—of all afflictions. With an ongoing devotion to draw forth this inherent disposition, the next stage of samyama can also transpire.

Dhyana

Dhyana comes from the Sanskrit roots *dhi*, meaning "receptacle," "design," "mind," "intellect," or "reflection," and *yana*, meaning "moving," "going," or "vehicle." It is regarded as the principle state of meditation, beyond concentration. It is reflected in a state of held equanimity and neutral awareness, without distraction. Dhyana may also refer to the level of the witness mind—a direct observation without any contrived thought. Here, the mind is truly steady and still. Awareness unfolds from the spiritual heart rather than the mental faculty (as in dharana). It is a gateway to the first stage of samadhi. The essence of this is revealed in Patanjali's Yoga Sutras:

> HRDAYE CHITTASAMVIT || 3.35 ||
>
> *(By performing saṃyama) on the heart, knowledge of the mind (is achieved).*[24]

Practically speaking, stillness does not denote meditation. Hopefully, this was made clear through the elaboration on dharana. There are practices that create an ideal environment that is conducive to allowing a state of meditation to arise. However, meditation is not a practice, per se. The techniques help to get us to meditation as dhyana, which is a state of being. The mind is no longer involved. Dhyana takes us deep into our individual consciousness, into the heart. We become one with the object of concentration. It dissolves. Only a vibration remains. There is the presence of an eternal principle of reverence and love for all of existence. Meditation as a *technique*—which is how it is mostly portrayed outside of the yoga traditions of India—does not reflect this distinction of dhyana. Interestingly, the Buddhist definition also differs from the yogic one.

Dhyana is a mystical aspect of yoga. It is not practical or overtly tangible. It cannot be intellectualized. Through stable detachment and dispassion (both of which are elements of vairagya), we can become receptive to this somewhat elusive, penultimate state that leads us to Patanjali's final limb, samadhi.

Samadhi

The final aspect of samyama, *samadhi*, translates to "accomplishment," "conclusion," "completion," "union," "intense absorption," "profound meditation," or "abstract meditation." Many suggest it is a state of transcendence or liberation. According to Patanjali's Yoga Sutras, there are multiple stages or levels of samadhi. This indicates how refined the condition can be.

The first stage is *samprajnata* samadhi. Also called *savikalpa* samadhi, simply speaking it conveys samadhi with some kind of object or "seed" for meditation. It is composed of *savitarka* (deliberation on a perceptible object) or *savichara* (reflection on the subtle aspect of an object that is not perceived by the senses). Or it is accompanied by *sananda* (a sattvic awareness of the state of bliss and ecstasy whereby savitarka and savicara have been dissolved or transcended) and *sasmita* (a concentration only on the sense of I-ness). In samprajnata samadhi, there is still a sense of ego and no loss of identity. But the identity expands temporarily into Supreme consciousness. The mind is conscious of the existence of spirit.

Asamprajnata samadhi is the second stage, also called *nirvikalpa* samadhi. It implies samadhi "without seed," or without an object. This higher state again is without ego. It is a realm where our samskaras and karmas are dissolved. There is no sense of time, only timelessness. Asamprajnata leads to a direct experience of purusha, or ever-present consciousness. Our latent vasanas are evaporated. It is a temporary state, and therefore one that we can "come down" from and continue to operate in the world.

Sahaja (meaning "natural") samadhi is when the state of the aforementioned asamprajnata samadhi is maintained throughout daily activity. It is certainly a more advanced and enigmatic state. Those engrossed in sahaja samadhi radiate a divine grace. They uphold an indescribable yet palpable luminosity.

Finally, *dharmamegha* samadhi eradicates any remaining samskaras or karmas. When this "cloud of virtue" dawns, the highest knowledge is attained. As a result, there is a cessation of the effects of the three gunas. It is experienced when there is an inherent loss of any desire to even know God or transcendence. It arises when even the most minute effort is dissolved. This is the highest state of the jivanmukta, a liberated and free being who still maintains their physical vessel.

There are other Sanskrit terms used across yogic teachings and traditions that bear a semblance to *samadhi*. They are *moksha*, *kaivalya*, and *nirvana*. These exalted states can all mean the same thing and also differ, depending on the text and school of philosophy. These heightened levels are attained usually while the physical body remains alive. They can also be experienced at the time of—and correlate to—one's physical death and liberation from that particular cycle of birth. These terms can also relate to complete freedom from samsara, meaning that when one dies there is no rebirth.

We learned a little about moksha in chapter three. Moksha is mentioned across a number of Vedic texts. When attained, it is an experience of the complete, limitless self. It comes with an inner and psychological freedom. Again, the Sanskrit word can translate to "eternal emancipation," "liberation," "death," or "release from worldly existence." Moksha is a release from suffering and samsara. Claimed to be a state of perfection, moksha is reflected in Self-realization. It can also relate to the enlightenment that coincides with—or potentially catalyzes—death. *Mumukshutva* is an early prelude to moksha. It is the seed planted through a conscious desire to attain this highest goal.

The fourth and final chapter of Patanjali's Yoga Sutras pertains to the state of kaivalya. It is concerned with the liberation, separation, or "detachment" from prakriti and a union with the Supreme. Kaivalya is deemed the ultimate goal, which is a constant state of undivided consciousness, of permanent liberation. This "emancipated" state is the heightened awareness that separates oneself from the material world to merge with the ultimate reality or truth. It is the "isolation" of purusha from prakriti. Oneness with Brahman is kaivalya. It could be said that kaivalya is the highest attainment of samadhi, where one is liberated from any bondage with the world.

The term *kaivalya* is used most commonly within the Samkhya school of philosophy. In chapter 43 of the much-loved text *Autobiography of a Yogi*, Sri Yukteswar Giri explains to his disciple, Yogananda, how desire is an "adhesive force by which all three bodies are held together."[25] These three bodies are the traya sharira, as touched on in chapter two. The desire Yukteswar speaks of is that which limits our capacity to reach the highest attainment of freedom. He goes on to emphasize, "The power of unfulfilled desires is the root of all man's slavery."[26]

Nirvana is a term used primarily in Buddhism. Synonymous with (but not quite the same as) moksha and kaivalya, nirvana is a state that can also be attained during one's lifetime. *Parinirvana* is the expression used when someone who has died has achieved nirvana—whether at death or prior. Nirvana relates to the concept of salvation and the cessation of samsara. Those who attain nirvana are freed from the suffering that maintains the cycle of birth and death. They are able to sustain uninterrupted peace. With nirvana, the pattern of rebirth terminates. The Sanskrit word translates to "blown out," "extinguished," "cessation," "calmed," and "deceased." It is regarded as the highest goal of most Buddhist traditions. The subtle difference between it and moksha or kaivalya is the concept of self. Moksha and kaivalya are seen as states that merge individual consciousness with the Supreme consciousness. In contrast, nirvana is a state where one dissolves any concept of consciousness. It is an obliteration ("extinction") of any sense of a higher Supreme being or consciousness. It is suggested to be an awareness devoid of absolutely anything.

There are clear parallels with each of these terms that have been given to the state of liberation or enlightenment. This further reiterates the complex layers of the tapestry of yoga. Ultimately, excess intellectualization inhibits our progress. Labels do not hold any value once we are immersed in the higher states of yoga. As always, the only way out is through. We must immerse in the practice and techniques to truly understand where we are going. While it is useful, intellectual knowledge will only take us so far. The following passage from the Bhagavad Gita sums up the essence of this clarity perfectly:

> YATROPARAMATA CHITTAM NIRUDDHAM YOGASEVAYA |
> YATRA CHAIVATMANATMANAM PASHYANNATMANI TUSHYATI || 6.20 ||
>
> In the still mind, in the depths of meditation, the Self reveals itself. Beholding the Self by means of the Self, an aspirant knows the joy and peace of complete fulfillment.[27]

The nectar of yoga lies within the direct experience. To find solace in the Supreme Reality we must embrace the dedication and unwavering devotion required to take us there, whether in this lifetime or many. May we find rest in the abode of the heart.

CONTEMPLATIONS

Which of the various yamas and niyamas do I uphold in my daily life, and which could I cultivate?

What was my understanding of asana before, and what is it now?

How could my yoga practice be more conducive to introspection and the development of subtle states of awareness?

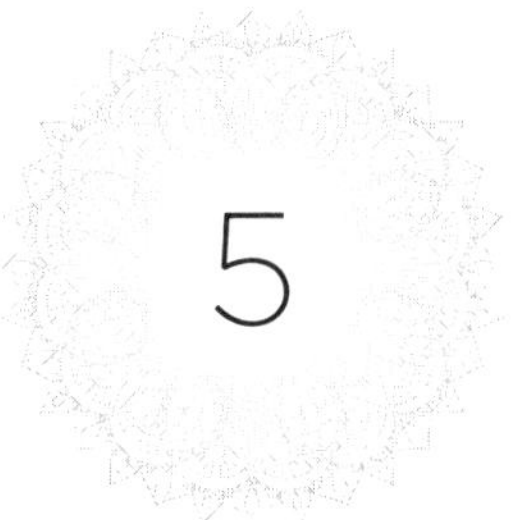

5

THE LANGUAGE OF YOGA

ACROSS ALL SPIRITUAL TRADITIONS and religions around the world, great emphasis is placed on pertinent texts, scriptures, and teachings. Within this is an incredible depth of reverence held for language and, even more specifically, for certain words or sounds. Consider *amen* as an example found in the Bible. Even the New Testament stresses this sentiment:

> In the beginning was the Word, and the Word was with God, and the Word was God.[28]

Deemed sacred and purifying, the study of traditional yoga shastras is believed to reveal the highest knowledge. Rich with meaning and beautiful in sound, these texts are believed to have a direct benefit on the physical body and the mind. The sacred scriptures presented here—and many more—are composed with either sutras, mantras, shlokas, or *stotras* (also called *stutis*). All are a wellspring of invaluable wisdom as explained here:

SUTRA: As in Patanjali's Yoga Sutras or Vatsyayana's *Kama Sutra*, these are compact statements that are "threaded" together to expound certain teachings.

MANTRA: As detailed in chapter four, these are consecrated Sanskrit words, statements, or sounds used to concentrate the mind and reach higher states.

SHLOKA: A rhythmic verse or hymn, or words arranged in a particular meter.

STOTRA: An elaborate verse in praise of someone or something; multiple shlokas put together make a stotra. Stotras are named based on the number of shlokas they contain.

Sanskrit and Sound

Lord Shiva is believed to have produced the very first sound, or *nada*—that being the creation of the universe itself. Therefore, it is not surprising that the Sanskrit language is sometimes believed to have emerged from Shiva's two-headed drum, the damaru. The drum represents the pulsing rhythm of life.

While Sanskrit is no longer a widely spoken language in the conversational sense, it is one of the most commonly used ancient languages in the world. Said to be the main language of yoga, it is regarded as a vehicle for the history and ancient culture of India. However, rightly argued, many feel that the ancient Dravidian languages may have just as much relevance to the traditions of India, including yoga. In this context, *Dravidian* refers to a collection of languages from South India that long predate Sanskrit. If we refer back to chapter one of this book, it is evident that Sanskrit evolved initially in North India due to the nomadic Indo-Aryan communities that slowly amalgamated into society. Regarded as a classical language just as Greek and Latin are, Sanskrit was possibly influenced by other ancient languages, and Dravidian could have been one of them. Interestingly, many English words appear to have origins in Sanskrit roots, such as *shampoo* (Hindi: *champo*; Sanskrit: *chapayati*) and *candy* (Sanskrit: *khanda*).

To truly know and understand this "language of the gods," Sanskrit requires perhaps lifetimes of study. From the root word, *samskrta*, which means "perfected," "well engineered," "refined," or "ornamented," Sanskrit is often regarded as the language, or sound, of the universe itself (*shabda-brahman*). As we unravel the root word further, we come to both *sama* and *kr*. *Kr* is one of the most common root sounds in Sanskrit. It generally means "to do." *Krita* means "done" or "made." *Sama*, meaning "same" and "even," implies doing something in a balanced way.

The Sanskrit language was originally passed on orally. A depth of listening, called *shruti*, ensured the language and teachings were well integrated into a person's mind. Panini, a great Indian grammarian, formally codified the language of Sanskrit in his book *Ashtadhyayi*. No doubt partly thanks to his work, the language is still alive and well across India and the globe today. Sanskrit not only has been used as a spoken language historically, but it also continues today in storytelling, performing arts, chanting, and of course through the instructions of modern, transnational yoga. The sentiment of the great value placed on the spoken language of Sanskrit (alongside Dravidian languages) within the Indic traditions is expressed the words of Swami Dayananda Saraswati: "The greatest musical instrument given to a human being is the voice."

Sanskrit is the language of the Vedas. The oldest known text written in Sanskrit is the Rigveda. This Vedic Sanskrit developed over time into Classical Sanskrit, which is very likely due to the influential systematization by Panini. The most notable differences between them are in structure and grammar, but there are more. Despite the organization of Sanskrit, it is important to reiterate that Sanskrit words generally have multiple or even numerous meanings. The translation or interpretation of any given word will have much to do with the context of the text and the way it is being used in a sentence (its syntax). Nonetheless, while scholars often can agree on overarching sentiments of the various texts and scriptures they are dedicated to decoding, their exact translations almost always differ in their word-by-word breakdown. Texts are often translated by academic approach. They can also be transmitted from the standpoint of a devotee or practitioner of a certain lineage. In this case, the language is conveyed with another type of insight, with a particular *bhava* (mood), and often greater symbolism or metaphor.

Nowadays, Sanskrit is most commonly written in a script called Devanagari. The word *devanagari* translates to "of the city of the gods." And perhaps unsurprisingly, Sanskrit got the name *devabhasha*, implying that it is so perfected that it is worthy of communication with the gods. This alludes to the importance of pronunciation and articulation, although there are subtle variations of pronunciation across India depending on the region. Heavily emphasized in mantra traditions, accuracy is incredibly valuable, if not essential. It is believed that Sanskrit was created as a means to generate a vibration within oneself, as a way to more effectively connect to that which one is focused on. Sanskrit in the form of mantra is said to generate sound patterns to promote states of mind that enable one to connect more easily and directly with a deity.

No doubt Sanskrit was guarded closely as a language. This is considered beneficial by some, and it is now a means to be transported into the past. Simultaneously, it thereby brings the past immediately into the present moment with the right awareness.

The Sanskrit word *pranava* refers to the mystical, sacred syllable of OM. OM is regarded as the primordial, foundational sound of the cosmos, an endless cosmic background hum or pulsation. It represents the emergence of prakriti from purusha—the motion of spirit. Also called *omkara*, it may well be the most important symbol, syllable, and sound within the yoga tradition. OM is often written as AUM. Just as the visual OM symbol has much hidden meaning, these letters of AUM also represent immense depth of insight. Here are a few of the most common attributes:

The A corresponds to creation, Brahma, the guna of rajas, and the waking state called *jagrat*.

The U corresponds to preservation, Vishnu, the sattva guna, and the dreaming state called *svapna*.

The M corresponds to destruction, Shiva, the guna of tamas, and the sleeping state called *sushupti*.

The bindu, dot, or silence after OM is associated with *gunatita*, that which is beyond the three gunas and therefore beyond the three levels of consciousness, a state called *turiya*.

It is worth noting that, within *some* traditions and lineages, any kind of recitation of the pranava mantra is reserved for only those who intend to renounce worldly life. This includes both verbal speaking and chanting of OM, along with any internal recitation. This may be surprising, given how incredibly routine it is to see, read, and chant this most sacred syllable in the present-day transnational yoga setting. With this perspective, it could be suggested that a householder is best served by abstaining from frequently engaging with the pranava until latter stages of life. Simultaneously, this could be disputed given the belief that all mantras (and the manifest world) arise out of OM and therefore OM is ever-present. Sadly, the visual "symbol" of OM—which is simply comprised of the Sanskrit letters of AUM—is often misappropriated. On the other end of the spectrum, many global yoga teachers and studios outside of India today completely avoid the pranava (visually and verbally) with an argument that it creates inaccessibility. Perhaps if OM were understood in greater depth, especially through sampradaya, there would be an awe and reverence toward it so that OM would be upheld in its rightful place.

Ultimately, Sanskrit syllables and words were created to produce *nada* (a sound vibration) within the speaker. This was to assist people in connecting more profoundly to the object or person they were verbally communicating with. Every time we speak, we create new karma, whether positive or negative. Hence, engaging in regular, extended periods of *mauna* (silence) is emphasized in the various Indic traditions, including Vedic, Buddhist, and Jain. This could be as simple as spending one day per week in silence (Saturday, which is ruled by Saturn, is most preferable). Mauna generally involves not only abstaining from verbal speech, but also avoiding other types of communication such as engaging in TV watching, social media, writing, gesturing, and the like. It is a real withdrawal, reducing new impressions on the mind. Alternatively, one could commit to a period of *vipashyana* (more commonly known as *vipassana*) on a silent retreat for approximately three to ten consecutive days annually. Or one could observe Mauni Amavasya, an annual day of silence in the Vedic calendar that falls on a particular dark moon date.

The Tamil sage Bhagavan Sri Ramana Maharshi (1879–1950) eloquently indicates the profound value of silence and mauna throughout his recorded talks, now published in multiple beloved books. Here is an example of his transformative guidance:

> That state which transcends speech and thought is *mouna*; it is meditation without mental activity. Subjugation of the mind is meditation: deep meditation is eternal speech. Silence is ever-speaking; it is the perennial flow of "language." It is interrupted by speaking; for words obstruct this mute language. Lectures may entertain individuals for hours without improving them. Silence, on the other hand, is permanent and benefits the whole of humanity. . . . By silence, eloquence is meant. Oral lectures are not so eloquent as silence. Silence is unceasing eloquence. It is the best language. There is a state when words cease and silence prevails.[29]

There are four types, or levels, of mauna, most commonly referenced in the Yoga Vasishtha:

VAC MAUNA: Silence of verbal speech.

INDRIYA MAUNA: Silence of the senses through pratyahara and meditation, for example.

KASHTHA MAUNA: A very strict level of silence that includes the first two levels, but also any other method of communication, such as journaling, writing, reading, gestures, and screen time.

SUSHUPTA MAUNA: Silence that is experienced in deep, dreamless sleep.

Similarly, there are four types or degrees of human speech, according to the Vedas. They are as follows, from the gross to the most subtle, or pure:

VAIKHARI: Ordinary verbal speech, associated with the past, present, and future.

MADHYAMA: This is internal dialogue that is verbalized but not spoken out loud. Also known as our internal monologue, it is the inner voice that questions and evaluates.

PASHYANTI: Here words are no longer formulated in any way, but there is a perceptible clarity of intention.

PARA: Beyond all desire and objects, this is the most subtle and highest level of pure intention summoned from Source, free from any adulteration.

In Sanskrit, the word for "speech" is *vac.* Vac is also the name of the Vedic goddess who is a personification of speech. She is believed to endow poets, singers, rishis, and the like with her qualities. Possessing them with her energy and expression, they are her vehicles. The goddess Vac is said to be the mother of the Veda. In later literature, we see her affiliated with Saraswati, who is the goddess of learning, art, music, knowledge, speech, and wisdom.

All of the manifest world has sprung forth from the most subtle of the five elements. That is akasha, or the space element. This element is related to the *sot-indriya*, the hearing faculty, and therefore our capacity to be receptive to *shabdaguna* (sound). In the same light, it is related to one of the jnanendriyas (organs of sense perception)—that of the ears, called *shrotrendriya.* The jnanendriyas are regarded as faculties of perception and knowledge acquisition. Sound then becomes more tangible when expressed through the mouth via speech, which is considered one of the *karmendriya* (organs of action) called *vaktattva.* Both sound and verbal speech are enlivened only through the presence of prana. Imagine the moment a baby is birthed into the world. They gasp to take their first breath of air and fill their lungs with this prana for the first time. The infant then goes on to make their first vocal expression of sound. This, in some sense, resembles and symbolizes the seemingly miraculous manifestation of all that is.

The Vedas and Upanishads

The root of the Sanskrit word *veda* comes from *vid*, which means "to know" or "to understand." In this context, it implies revered or sacred knowledge. The Vedas are a vast body of work that are often likened to mystical poetry. They are understood to speak generally of a systematic spiritual ascent of human beings and about the laws of truth.

Eventually written down in *Vedic* Sanskrit, these high-caliber texts were initially divinely revealed to the Rishis (or seers), who never went on to claim ownership of the knowledge. Through the deep meditation and spiritual discipline of the Rishis, this wisdom of the Vedas was received and passed on through lineage. It was Maharishi Krishna Dvaipayana, also known as Veda Vyasa, who formally compiled all the *apaurusheya* (authorless knowledge that is not of humankind) and classified it into the Vedas we know today.

The Vedas teach of the interconnectedness of the cosmos, governed by laws of truth that are executed by the divine functionaries—the deities—in charge of this current manifestation. For those who grow up immersed in the Vedic teachings, this resonance of eternal truth is heard and felt, thereby guiding them to live more intelligently.

Naturally, the Vedas were originally transmitted by oral tradition. Even today, when someone comes to study the Vedas, the approach is via sound rather than trying to intellectually translate the mantras and hymns. Specifically, this is through listening to and reciting the mantras over and over. As a result, when we come to eventually decode the translations—after generous listening and regular recitation—the mantras have already revealed to us a degree of meaning so we can realize them on an experiential level. We can internalize their meaning far more easily.

Each of the texts teaches us a wealth of spiritual knowledge and knowledge of everyday life. This includes health, education, ecology, economics, governance, harmonious living, establishment of inner peace, techniques of ritual, practical mantras, and more. They teach us that everything in life is divine, that there is no need to become a renunciant necessarily. Everything in life is a precious resource, and we have the gift to be able to create a relationship with the divine through everything around us. Interestingly, within the Vedas, we learn of multiple *rishikas* (female seers) as well as *brahmavadinis* (female teachers).

The Vedas are broken down into four separate texts, as mentioned in chapter one:

RIGVEDA: This is the oldest text and is grouped into ten *mandala* (circles, divisions, or books). It hosts a compilation of *sukta* (hymns) and descriptive words of praise. These hymns describe properties of the natural elements around us and personify their forms.

SAMAVEDA: In a simplistic sense, this text contains an emphasis on song. The verses are sung by priests during public worship.

They are uttered to a set tune or melody. The Samaveda pulls many of the same hymns from the Rigveda. This text is often regarded as the origin of the field of *samgita* (music and performative arts) within India.

YAJURVEDA: This text emphasizes the power of ritual. It offers instructions on how to conduct various types of rituals associated with promoting the well-being of humankind. It shares the formulas for the actions performed in front of the yajna, or holy fire. The Yajurveda is twofold. The Krishna Yajurveda is characterized by a mixture of mantra and *brahmana* and is more popular in South India. The Shukla Yajurveda clearly separates the two and is more popular in North India.

ATHARVAVEDA: The youngest of the four texts, the Atharvaveda represents various rites and medicines used to address both mental and physical ailments. In one sense it presents traditional folk healing, but in another, some believe the various formulas represent magic. The Atharvaveda has long been a source text that speaks to marriage and also to death—cremation more specifically. The text is regarded as very practical, given it addresses how to handle life at the physical level of existence. It offers guidance on dealing with discomfort, how to acquire wealth (of all kinds), and how to disseminate it appropriately.

Across all four texts there is mention of many deities. Some of the main ones are Agni, Surya, Vayu, Indra, Mitra, Varuna, Saraswati, Bhaga, Soma, and Durga.

Each text is broken down into four components. It is believed that there are six additional fields of study, called *vedanga*, that assist us in understanding these four components:

SAMHITA: A compilation of realized hymns devoted to the forces of nature and staying in alignment with them.

BRAHMANA: Explanations of how to put the hymns to practical use, usually through elaborate ritual.

ARANYAKA: Various internal observances one needs to follow, and themes uncovered through meditation.

UPANISHAD: The most well-known part of the Vedas, these are poetic footnotes that capture the essence of each of the texts and teach us the true nature of reality.

These four components are sometimes layered over the four ashramas (see chapter three), with each having a greater emphasis and value across the stages of one's life. For example, the Samhita section is more relevant to someone in the brahmacharya ashrama, during their educational upbringing and height of studentship. The Brahmana section is pertinent to the householder or during the grhastha period, whereby one is expected to put the learning of the Samhita into practical use to uplift society. As one slowly withdraws later in life, during the vanaprastha period, spiritual pursuits are to be strongly engaged. Finally, the sannyasa ashrama embraces the essence of the Upanishad components to further one's renouncing of the world and continued search for absolute truth.

Given the context of this book, the Upanishads deserve further elaboration. As touched on briefly in chapter one, the Rigveda is where we uncover the first use of the word *yoga*. Yet it is not until we dive into the Upanishads that we see the word used in a more practical and relevant context. The word *upanishad*, as earlier established, means "to sit down near." This references the act of sitting near the guru to receive teachings about the true nature of reality. To have our delusions destroyed. There are both major (at least ten) and minor Upanishads, with the belief that there are 108 in total, although that number has been challenged. Regardless of their individual importance, some Upanishads are very small in size, with only a few verses. Others are huge.

Out of the ten or so major Upanishads, most commonly it is the *Mandukya*—from the Atharvaveda—that is regarded as the most important. The Mandukya is a very accessible composition, given it is only twelve verses long. It delves into the syllable of AUM, the four states of consciousness (related to the invaluable practice of yoga nidra), and also the concept of *atman*, the eternal essence of each individual. Alternatively, the *Ishopanishad* (*Isha Upanishad*) from the Yajurveda is held in primary esteem. It is one of the most important Upanishad texts within Vedanta philosophy. Comprised of seventeen to eighteen verses, the

Ishopanishad addresses the conflict between pursuing a spiritual path of direct knowledge and renunciation, versus a path of the householder and the resulting accumulation of karma. It emphasizes the value of embracing a virtuous life and the pursuit of true knowledge—that which leads to the understanding of true unity and of the imperishable highest Self.

The six vedangas that aid us in understanding the four noted sections of each Veda are as follows:

SHIKSHA: Focuses on the rules of Sanskrit pronunciation, such as stress, phonetics, accent, and more.

CHANDAS: Focuses on the poetic meter of each verse.

VYAKARANA: Focuses on correct grammar to properly express ideas.

NIRUKTA: Focuses on clarifying and explaining the meaning of words based on their context of use (etymology).

KALPA: Focuses on establishing standard procedures and proper mantra application for rites and rituals, plus an individual's duties across varying stages of life.

JYOTISHA: Focuses on the study of time and light through the lens of astronomy and astrology.

Each of the four Vedas—Rigveda, Yajurveda, Samaveda, and Atharvaveda—has been ascribed a subsystem of knowledge. Called *upaveda*, these are born out of the revelations presented within each Veda. Ayurveda is associated with both the Rigveda and the Atharvaveda. Dhanurveda—the study of warfare and archery—is ascribed to the Yajurveda. Gandharvaveda—the study of the arts, including music, dance, drama, and aesthetics—is connected to the Samaveda. Lastly, Arthashastram—the study of all kinds of wealth and prosperity—is associated with the Atharvaveda. However, this last upaveda is argued, and some instead include Sthapatyaveda, the science of architecture (mostly related to temple design specifically), which is linked to the more commonly known Vastu.

Some give prominence to a fifth Veda that also holds immense importance. Usually this is claimed to be Veda Vyasa's Mahabharata, or the

Ramacharitamanasa (based on the Ramayana) by sage Tulsi Das, or otherwise the *Natya Shastra* by Bharat Muni (this is a heavily valued text within the arts communities of dance and drama in India).

The Vedas have no doubt influenced Indian culture and the yoga tradition, even as we know it today. They have directly informed Vedanta, Tantra, and classical yoga in varying ways. The teachings of the Veda are eternal in nature and thereby intended to transcend any association with religion or dogma. Despite some subtle indications of the nature of society at the time when they were revealed and initially disseminated, the essence of the Vedas has value for everyone at any time.

Bhagavad Gita

The "Song of God," the Bhagavad Gita is a remarkable 700-verse text highly revered within India. Part of the much larger epic the Mahabharata, the Gita is a dialogue (*samvada* in Sanskrit) between Prince Arjuna and his charioteer guide, Krishna—whom Arjuna later discovers is one of the incarnations and avatars of Lord Vishnu. Considered the "jewel" of the Mahabharata (as it is found in the center of the text), this scripture has also been highly regarded within the global yoga community. As mentioned in chapter one, the Bhagavad Gita offers numerous meanings for the word *yoga*. One of the most common translations suggests "skillful action" in the world. Many hold the text in such high esteem they propose that there is little necessity in studying any other scriptural texts, as the Gita has everlasting relevance to all. It is said to contain everything one may need to know.

The setting for the dialogue between Krishna and Arjuna is a battlefield. Arjuna is confronted with the conflicting need to face his duty to fight in the war in front of him and his affection for his extended family and community who are standing on both sides. He is troubled and depressed. The fight is for the kingdom, after decades of dispute. Arjuna, being the greatest archer and *kshatriya* (warrior), is destined to face his duty, his dharma. He is dismayed by the reality of killing his relatives and asks his friend Krishna what to do. As a result, Krishna decides to lecture Arjuna—sometimes quite assertively—with sublime guidance to ensure that order and justice are upheld. His abrasive approach fails to move Arjuna enough to act, so Krishna adopts a far more reassuring tone while presenting the wisdom of yoga as a means to engaging within the world.

Krishna continues to urge Arjuna toward dispassion and non-attachment to outcomes and rewards when engaged in worldly duty. He encourages Arjuna to relinquish and transcend all desires. Equanimity, after all, is one of Krishna's definitions of yoga. A key message of the text is to move toward a life where one is selflessly acting in the world. Rather than avoiding taking action, or otherwise clinging to the fruits of our action, we are to engage with the world detached from the outcomes and results. One may then consider inaction altogether, but this ultimately has a selfish intent and inevitably leads to karmic ramifications.

Next, we witness Krishna guiding the warrior Arjuna toward a stilling of the mind. This is with the intent to assist Arjuna in connecting to his higher intellect and buddhi mind. It is here we read of sensory withdrawal as another example of yoga. Through a mastery of the mind and senses that results in emotional neutrality, Krishna affirms to Arjuna that there is no dishonor in taking right action to bring everything back into divine order. Eventually, Arjuna comes to realize that his friend, the charioteer Krishna, is someone far greater. Through long contemplation and rumination, acknowledging his fundamental concern for the nature of being human, Arjuna commits to Krishna as his student.

Krishna goes on to further teach Arjuna the path to freedom from turmoil, to tranquility, to true knowledge, to yoga. Krishna implores Arjuna to have unwavering faith and wholehearted devotion toward him. He tells Arjuna that it is through Bhakti yoga that one can fast-track one's way to Self-realization. We read of Arjuna's yearning to know more directly of Krishna's divinity. The Lord reveals himself in an astonishing and monumental mystical display, which Arjuna finds overwhelming and almost incomprehensible.

Throughout the discourse, Arjuna matures and gathers wisdom to move forward with greater clarity and certainty. Arjuna comes to see through the illusion of his humanness. He perceives all the god-like qualities one is meant to embody, and the immense value of service—selfless service being the motivation behind all action. Krishna drives home the invaluable direction of embracing one's dharma instead of renouncing the world—unless, of course, that is your genuine duty.

Praised as a form of the divine mother, the Bhagavad Gita sheds light on many paths toward yoga, the most important being Karma yoga, Jnana yoga, Bhakti yoga, and Raja yoga. Relevant to any spiritual aspirant, it has a universal appeal, as it does not present or align with one particular school of philosophy exclusively. This "divine song" illuminates the essential worth of pursuing service in the world through the lens of our unique dharma, all while renouncing attachment to the fruits of our actions. It sheds light on the three gunas and the fabric of existence.

Despite its dramatic nature, the Gita is a timeless and practical manual for everyday life. Significantly, it is sometimes taught through a very specific understanding that can be incredibly useful and powerful. This is that the Bhagavad Gita is happening *within* ourselves. It is our own internal battle with our illusions, ignorance, desires, and attachments—a seemingly endless internal battle between the darkness and the light. So, while the text clearly offers the reader many practical ways to pursue a virtuous path of yoga, another seed full of potential is to study the text as though all the characters and dialogue are a part of oneself. This is beautifully expressed by Pujya Swami Dayananda Saraswati:

> *In the Gita you will find yourself;*
> *The self hitherto unknown but sought after,*
> *The self that is strangely missed and searched for,*
> *The self that you love to be,*
> *That you are.*[30]

An important addition here is to highlight the highly valued commentary on the Bhagavad Gita, usually called the *Jnaneshwari*. Also titled the *Bhavartha Deepika*, this interpretation was written by poet, philosopher, and yogi Sant Dnyaneshwar (born 1275 C.E.). His rendition reflects a strong affinity toward Advaita Vedanta and Bhakti yoga. Compared to the Bhagavad Gita's 700 verses, the Jnaneshwari is notably expanded and comprises around 9,000 verses. Originally written in the Marathi language, it weaves through mention of a number of various Indian philosophical systems and texts. An accessible English translation is one compiled by Swami Kripananda.

Again, the Bhagavad Gita is only a small part of the far greater "poem," the Mahabharata, attributed to the sage Vyasa. The Mahabharata is structured in a way that it holds stories within the greater story. Spoiler alert: the epic ends with the death of Lord Krishna, marking the beginning of the age of Kali Yuga (not to be confused with, or directly correlated to, the goddess Kali (KAH-lee), whose name is pronounced with a longer "a" sound).

Yoga Yajnavalkya

Often claimed to be a Hatha yoga text, the Yoga Yajnavalkya is in the form of a conversation between enlightened sage Yajnavalkya and his wife, philosopher Gargi Vachaknavi. Her involvement is historically significant. Given the rare connection of women to yoga, this text is encouraging for any female student. In fact, a few of the verses are suggested to be addressed to women only. Containing an accessible 504 verses, the Yajnavalkya has no confirmed time of composition. Some propose it belongs somewhere around the second to fifth century C.E., on the basis that Yajnavalkya's teachings appear in later texts. Others suggest it was composed around the twelfth to thirteenth century C.E. Regardless of this continuing question among scholars and Indologists, the text certainly provides immense value to any practitioner of yoga.

The Yoga Yajnavalkya has not received the same worthy attention among students and teachers of yoga as other texts. Yet, it has significantly informed several well-known works, such as the Hatha Pradipika from the fifteenth century C.E. and many of the Yoga Upanishads. It has been *suggested* that the Yoga Yajnavalkya was, at one stage, far more notable in society than the Yoga Sutras of Patanjali.

Beautifully, the sage Yajnavalkya evidently has deep respect, reverence, and adoration for his wife, as displayed all throughout the text. Upon Gargi's request—and in the presence of other revered sages—he explains the principles and practices of yoga, with emphasis on pranayama, the subtle body, and meditation. A few asanas are also woven through as preliminary preparations for the principle techniques. It is worth noting that, of the eight postures mentioned, none are standing poses. Seven are seated postures, and one is an arm balance.

The Yoga Yajnavalkya is clearly aligned with Advaita Vedantic, nondual thought. However, despite its clear Vedic influence, the text also alludes to techniques and studies of the Tantras. The text speaks to prana and its movement through the system of nadis (nadi shuddhi), alongside the activation of kundalini. It outlines the limbs, or auxiliaries, of yoga, with slight variance to those in Patanjali's Yoga Sutras. It is in this text that we read the descriptions of ten yamas and ten niyamas, for example.

Through the detailed and sequential steps Yajnavalkya highlights, he teaches how to release bondage of the mind, how to move beyond (mental) enemies and eventually attain the experience of samadhi, or enlightenment. Various direct techniques are taught in the Yoga Yajnavalkya, alongside discerning clarifications around the various types of pratyahara (sensory withdrawal) and dhyana (meditation). Perhaps the most emphasis appears to be placed by Yajnavalkya on the diligent practice of pranayama, such as nadi shodhana, in addition to the internal recitation of the pranava mantra, OM. At the end of the text, as Yajnavalkya enters a state of samadhi, Gargi takes herself to the forest to live in solitude and adhere to the teachings laid out by her husband. This is an uncommon account of a woman evidently engaging in the practice of yoga.

There are only a couple of English translations of the Yoga Yajnavalkya, the more common being that by A. G. Mohan and the other from the Krishnamacharya Yoga Mandiram. It was deemed a very important text by Krishnamacharya himself during the twenthieth century, despite being commonly overlooked today. Overall, the Yoga Yajnavalkya aims to disclose the nature of yoga via an inward-moving practical path of virtuous observances, self-restraint, and techniques.

Yoga Vasishtha

The Yoga Vasishtha is a highly influential and pivotal text, typically attributed to sage and poet Valmiki, author of the epic poem the Ramayana. The full *brhat* (meaning "great" or "large") version contains well over 29,000 verses. A condensed version entitled *Laghu Yogavasishtha* contains 6,000 verses. The Sanskrit word *laghu* means "light," "short," and "easy to digest." The date of composition is unconfirmed and speculative. Depending on the scholar or lineage, it is most often claimed to be a text compiled somewhere around the sixth century C.E. Also called the *Vasishtha Ramayana*, the text is a dialogue between the sage Vasishtha and the young prince Rama. The illuminating discourse unveils deep stories and a wealth of timeless wisdom. Interestingly, where in the Bhagavad Gita we have God (specifically Vishnu in the form of Lord Krishna) who takes the role of teacher, with Arjuna as the student, in the Yoga

Vasishtha it is a human, Sage Vasishtha, who assumes the role of teacher to Lord Rama (another incarnation of Vishnu).

The text consists of six books or parts. Using an accessible English translation by Swami Venkatesananda as a basis, this section will discuss some of the key themes illumined in each. Part one ("Vairagya-prakaranam") of the Yoga Vasishtha begins with young Rama, who is only in his early teens, returning from a pilgrimage across India—a yatra that altered him physically, mentally, and spiritually. With the passing of time, his father's concern grows as the prince becomes more withdrawn and emaciated. One day, the king summons Rama to speak with him in the presence of many wise sages, such as Vishvamitra and, of course, Vasishtha. Rama finally reveals his disdain for the world. He declares his frustration over having no desire or attachment to any aspect of worldly life yet still experiencing misery. It becomes evident that he has come to a higher knowledge of the nature of reality. Simultaneously he is aware that he has not experienced the freedom he anticipated from perceiving the truth. Rama mentions the repetitive cycle of existence known as samsara. He scrutinizes the degradation of various stages of life and the delusion of time. Finally seeking guidance on how to free oneself from delusion, Rama falls silent.

Part two ("Mumukshu-vyavahara-prakaranam") opens with Sage Vishvamitra recognizing Rama's supreme wisdom. He urges Vasishtha to take on the role of instructing Rama so that he is reassured and confirmed in his insight. Sage Vasishtha goes on to clarify what is meant by self-effort and its value. Teaching Rama, he states that self-effort is based on a combination of keen study of scripture, guidance from one's teacher and, lastly, one's own efforts. He sheds light on "fate," illuminating the concept of samskara as the cause of all unexplained circumstances. Through this we are reminded that we can strengthen the pure latent tendencies within and utilize the present moment to resolve impure ones—those expressed by seemingly adverse experiences.

Vasishtha continues to disclose the four gatekeepers at the entrance to the "Realm of Freedom," or liberation. These are self-control, spirit of inquiry, contentment, and keeping good company. Elaborating, he explains that the eternal is attained only by the conquest of one's mind. Not via wealth, pilgrimage, or any ritual. Vasishtha emphasizes that self-control of the mind is the remedy for all sorrow. Inquiry is explained to be a direct looking into oneself, by asking "Who am I?" for example. He claims that this inquiry is the best remedy for samsara. To embody contentment one must renounce all craving and thereby maintain dispassion toward everything. Lastly, Sage Vasishtha highlights the necessity of keeping the regular company of wise persons. This endorsement for *satsanga* is a reminder to always be aware of our associations.

Part three ("Utpatti-prakaranam") is an exposition filled with a wealth of illuminating metaphors and stories. Over the course of a few days, Vasishtha describes the birth of all creation from a nondual perspective. Reiterating the importance of keeping good company (of holy persons), the study of scripture, and a renunciation of all craving, we come to learn the nature of *jíva*—the individual living soul. Vasishtha also advises the best text for scriptural study. He goes on to teach Rama about the mind, how it is the root of all suffering and the "unreal" manifest world. Part three also touches briefly on death, the relationship between the elements and senses, and also the three gunas: tamas, rajas, and sattva. Rama inquires into the mystery of time, of God, and how ignorance arises within. He asks questions that may naturally arise for the reader as a serious student on the path of yoga.

Part four ("Sthiti-prakaranam") continues with further nondualistic ideas. Vasishtha's discourse highlights the nature of the wise person. He emphasizes how, for enlightened ones, the body is regarded purely as a vehicle of wisdom for the liberation of the soul. Through further metaphors and stories, it is affirmed that all notions of unity or liberation only reinforce a dualistic state of mind. Vasishtha presses that these concepts simply pertain to the manifest "unreal" world. Therefore, they cease to exist in the realm of the infinite consciousness. We are again reminded to study scripture, and to do so with a teacher who has had a direct experience of the truth.

Vasishtha recounts several tales in part five ("Upashanti-prakaranam") that continue to promote his teachings thus far. Urging non-attachment by means of self-control, he alludes to the state of equanimity multiple times. Comparisons are made between the ignorant and the wise to highlight the origin of all suffering in the world. Rama again asks reasonable questions that inevitably arise on a course of deep inquiry. It is in part five that we see a greater emphasis on aspects of yoga that are seemingly more practical and commonly known today—these being the use of the pranava, mention of prana and apana vayu, pranayama, breath retentions, tongue placement (as in kechari mudra), withdrawal of the senses, yoga asana (in its true sense as a seated posture), mantra recitation, meditation, and simply the idea of "being" a yogi. Through the dialogue between Vasishtha and Rama, the state of mental quiescence is repeatedly accentuated as being of utmost importance to achieve the liberated state.

Part six ("Nirvana-prakaranam") is the final part of the Yoga Vasishtha, as we read of Rama moving into the state of enlightenment. Alive with another collection of stories that engage us, here the text culminates with further reminders that yoga is a transcendence of the mind, the supreme yoga being Self-knowledge gained through meditation. Guidance from Vasishtha becomes slightly more practical as we learn of more specifics within pranayama and the techniques of kumbhaka. It is reiterated that concepts and words such as "creation," "God," and "Brahman" are all part of the illusion that suggests duality. Clarity is shed on the distinction between being enlightened while still operating within the world and the physical body, and experiencing enlightenment that moves one into full transcendence of the physical body.

The essence of the Bhagavad Gita shines through at one point in part six. We additionally learn of the four stages of silence and of the three doshas. Although only small, there is a story that suggests the immense value of women on the spiritual path alongside men. Significantly, Vasishtha firmly reminds us that intellectual knowledge is not true knowledge, that it is still tied to dualism. To become firmly established in non-attachment, dispassion and awareness of the Supreme consciousness only are the goal.

Overall, the text offers us some insight into a very traditional path of yoga, in the truest sense of the word—one that takes us toward union with the infinite consciousness, beyond delusion and self-identification. Woven with subtle hints and clues, the Yoga Vasishtha reinforces the same teachings repeatedly throughout the changing lens of its timeless stories. Cherished by the Indian jivanmukta Ramana Maharshi, it both raises and answers questions that may emerge naturally on the path for those who seek depth through heartfelt inquiry.

Yoga Sutras of Patanjali

As touched on previously in chapter three, Patanjali's Yoga Sutras are regarded as the basis of one of the six darshanas, or schools of philosophy. Written in Sanskrit, the text is often used as an authoritative manual in modern yoga. This is despite the fact that it places extremely little emphasis on anything postural. The Yoga Sutras text has been translated and commentated on numerous times over many years. The result of this is that often it is presented through a changing lens. A positive outcome of such an approach is that it ensures the text has relevance to the present day. However, it can simultaneously dilute the original intent and essence of the text.

The Yoga Sutras of Patanjali are studied from both an academic viewpoint and also that of tradition or lineage. Due to this, we often see conflicting interpretations of certain teachings from Patanjali. The academic perspective has immense value but can be significantly more literal. Most commonly it is advised *not* to study the text from a purely intellectual position. Based on the teachings of Samkhya philosophy, the Yoga Sutras are often seen as principally—although certainly not entirely—supportive of an ascetic life. This collection is seen as a key text for the yogi (in the true sense of the word). This is in contrast to the other most popular yoga text, the Bhagavad Gita, which is presented as the ultimate text in the householder tradition. Nonetheless, there is no doubt that most of the Yoga Sutras' framework can be adapted and embraced to suit a householder of the modern, affluent world. In addition, Patanjali's treatise also reflects Upanishadic and Buddhist influence. So, although it is the basis of the Yoga school of philosophy it holds influence from diverse sources.

Who Patanjali was is inconclusive. Some believe the Yoga Sutras were written by the sage Patanjali, an avatar of Adishesha. There is another Patanjali, the linguist and grammarian, who wrote a commentary on Sanskrit around the second century B.C.E. There is also the Patanjali who was a medical authority who composed various Sanskrit medical texts. In addition, yet another Patanjali—a scholar who lived at a later time—wrote commentary on the revered Ayurvedic *Charaka-Samhita*. Many believe in there only being one Patanjali who assembled three specific texts on Sanskrit, Ayurveda, and yoga. It is he who is honored in the invocation recited at the beginning of any Iyengar or ashtanga yoga practice. A senior yoga teacher, Alan Finger,[31] proposed that the Patanjali who authored the Yoga Sutras may have also been a Tantrika.

Speculations aside, the Sanskrit word *sutra* comes from the root, *su*. Sutra means "thread." In this context it refers to a short, succinct, and condensed statement. The word *sutra* is used across titles of many Indian texts in diverse fields of study. Any sutra is designed to be unpacked. These pithy aphorisms are intentionally minimal, as they are traditionally used as a support to the custom of oral learning with an accomplished teacher. Depth of meaning cannot be grasped from just briefly reading through each compact statement. Woven together within Patanjali's acclaimed manual are 195 (or 196) sutras. Due to the large number of translations—and varied interpretations—it is generally recommended to study the Yoga Sutras alongside the traditional *bhashya* (commentary) from Veda Vyasa or Adi Shankaracharya. However, this may be realistic only for those who are adept in reading Sanskrit or who can access a teacher with this level of knowledge.

The text is broken up into four chapters, or padas. The Sanskrit word *pada* translates to "foot," "column," and "pillar." Each of these four feet upholds the body of work. Like four essential columns of a building, they each bear their own importance, and they are synergistic in value.

Entitled *Samadhi Pada*, chapter 1 opens with the following verse:

> ATHA YOGA-ANUSHASANAM || 1.1 ||

This first sutra is translated in multiple ways, as follows:

> Now the teachings of yoga are being explained.[32]
>
> In the Now, yoga happens.[33]
>
> Now, the teachings of yoga [are presented].[34]
>
> With humility (an open heart and mind), we embrace the sacred study of yoga.[35]

Even with the very first word, *atha*, already there is the potential to go beyond the obvious. Some interpret this "now" as implying something potentially hierarchical over other yogic texts. Others may think it simply suggests something of the present moment. However, other commentary attests to *atha* as being an auspicious beginning and equivalent to the use of OM. Thereby, the first sutra can be regarded as a prayer.

Patanjali goes on to define yoga through the renowned verse, sutra 1.2: yogash-chitta-vrtti-nirodha. This sutra is widely accepted as conveying that "yoga is the stilling of the changing states of the mind."[36] We learn of the five types of *vrtti* that are the mental fluctuations or changing states. These vrttis have the potential to be either beneficial or detrimental to a path of yoga. We are introduced to the well-known concepts of abhyasa (practice) and vairagya (dispassion) as the means of stilling these mental modifications. The two key variations of samadhi are brought to light: samprajnata and asamprajnata. Samadhi is the ultimate goal and technique to attain the state of kaivalya, which is expanded upon in chapter 4. *Samapatti* (sum-AH-puh-tee) is introduced as somewhat of a prerequisite to attaining samadhi. Samapatti is a state of utter equilibrium of the mind, accessed through dhyana, or meditation.

Chapter 2, *Sadhana Pada*, outlines Patanjali's practical pathway of kriya yoga and ashtanga yoga. Here, kriya yoga simply refers to the essential actions required to move into the ashtanga system and eventually attain samadhi. These are—according to Patanjali—tapas, svadhyaya, and Ishvarapranidhana. Also called raja yoga, the eight-limbed, systematic method of ashtanga yoga is often interpreted as a linear approach. Yet each step comes together to work cohesively with the next, without leaving any aspect behind, as one progresses along the path. While all eight steps are introduced here, this chapter of the Yoga Sutras expands on the first five limbs only (*bahiranga sadhana*). They are yama, niyama, asana, pranayama, and pratyahara. *Sadhana Pada* also discusses five kleshas as the main impediments—which can be weakened by the actions of kriya yoga—to reaching samadhi. Patanjali presses that these kleshas are the root of our karma, of the cycle of samsara (rebirth).

Chapter 3 is titled *Vibhuti Pada*. *Vibhuti* is a Sanskrit word that means "pervading," "powerful," and "expansion." It also refers to the sacred ash made from cow dung during rituals by devotees of Lord Shiva (which they then smear across the forehead and body, as Shiva himself is said to do). This chapter presents the final, far more internal three limbs of ashtanga yoga called *antaranga sadhana*. Simultaneously performed and held together, these three—dharana, dhyana, and samadhi—culminate in samyama.

However, *Vibhuti Pada* focuses more on the potential of attaining siddhis. These various achievements of power come with a clear warning, despite sometimes being viewed as magnificent fruits of yogic accomplishments. Patanjali repeatedly alludes to their nature of distracting one from the ultimate goal. Depending on how these somewhat elusive psychic powers are interpreted, a few of them are deemed relatively accessible for the dedicated practitioner. Unsurprisingly, on initial inquiry, the other siddhis will seem far-fetched to most practitioners. Regardless, we are reminded that, if they arise through our sadhana, the only way to proceed is to renounce them. In addition, the word *siddhi* is often believed to imply "perfection," that is, a certain perfection attained through the fulfillment of one's yoga practice.

Kaivalya Pada is the fourth and final pada of Patanjali's treatise. The chapter begins by listing various means to attaining the aforementioned siddhis:

> JANMAUSHADHI-MANTRA-TAPAH-SAMADHIJAH SIDDHAYAḤ || 4.1 ||

From varied commentators, its translation:

> Supernatural powers are obtained by birth, herbs, mantra, austerity, or samadhi.[37]
>
> One is either born with siddhis or they arise from using herbs, repeating mantras, mental focus and purification, and being in the state of Samadhi.[38]
>
> The mystic powers arise due to birth, herbs, mantras, the performance of austerity, and samadhi.[39]

In chapter 4, Patanjali also expands upon karma, samskaras, and time. He guides us on how to resolve or neutralize existing karma and also how to cease the generation of new karma. We learn the benefits of the highest form of discriminative insight, which in turn leads us toward a life lived with a pure consciousness that is beyond the duality of the mind. The Sanskrit word *kaivalya* literally translates to "isolation." In this context, the word may well relate to the perfect isolation or *separation* of consciousness from all forms of matter, that is, those that normally reside within the mind and our field of awareness. Patanjali intends to illuminate the process of becoming established in an awareness of the Seer. He attempts to describe our inherent cosmic nature, which is beyond all conditions and attributes. *Kaívalya* is also used to imply emancipation. In the simplest sense, chapter 4 concerns itself with shifting the mind from master to servant, accessing the freedom that arises when we know "our" true Self.

Patanjali's Yoga Sutras highlight a path of yoga that transcends a physical set of practices—certainly anything akin to what we commonly see today in mainstream postural yoga. Rather, he invites us into experiential wisdom. This can be further emphasized through the traditional approach of verbal Sanskrit sutra recitation—unlocking the essence of each sutra through sound. The sacred text has the potential to offer us greater awareness and deep transformation. It is important to remember that the Yoga Sutras, as one of the earliest Sanskrit yoga-related texts to be translated to English, has many varying interpretations across numerous respected scholars and revered teachers. As with all shastra, the teachings require in-depth contemplation, reflection, and an appreciation for the historical lens through which a text was complied. While the text evidently holds strong Samkhya influence, threads can be linked to other revered teachings, such as those within the Bhagavad Gita and various Upanishads.

Hatha Pradipika

An authoritative and hugely influential text, the Hatha Pradipika gives us a glimpse into the yogic techniques and practices that helped to shape modern yoga developments. Often known as the Hatha Yoga Pradipika, the title commonly translates to the "light," "lamp," or "illumination" on Hatha yoga. Compiled by the yogi Svatmarama in the early fifteenth century C.E., the treatise is divided into four key chapters that reveal a very practical approach and pathway toward the state of yoga. In fact, this significant Sanskrit shastra is a compilation of verses drawn from several earlier yoga-related texts. Because of this, when studied closely, there are some contradictions that can be observed within the text.

Many of the techniques within the Hatha Pradipika—especially those that are nonpostural—have been lost within modern transnational yoga. Even through the lens of studio classes named "hatha," the experience is devoid of any indication of the Hatha tradition. Despite this, the text has historically informed much of the modern yoga developments, even though, notably, none of the yoga postures mentioned in the Hatha Pradipika are standing poses. The approach that Svatmarama offers in the text begins with purifying the physical body. This is in essential preparation for the higher meditative techniques of Raja yoga. He presents a practical and systematic "stairway" toward the higher states of yoga. In terms of the physical practices, there is greater emphasis on pranayama (specifically kumbhaka) and mudra over the selection of asana. This is in spite of the fact that the Hatha Pradipika was the first in history to list as many asanas as it did (fifteen to be exact). As with most yogic texts, this exposition cryptically veils some of the teachings, as the writing is meant to be purely an aid and a supplement for the practitioner who is studying under the guidance of a masterful teacher. Many of the techniques require elaboration and caution.

Chapter 1 begins with salutations to Lord Shiva, often said to be the original yogi and disseminator of the Hatha *vidya* (knowledge or science). Svatmarama acknowledges the lineage, reciting many names of previous Hatha masters. He reminds the reader that the knowledge being passed on provides refuge and should be guarded to maintain its efficacy. The chapter then sheds light on the ideal environment for yoga, ethics to uphold, the yogic diet, and a selection of yoga postures. We are told of the ultimate asana one should engage in every day as a means to purify all of the nadis. Moderation of diet and general nonviolence are emphasized as the most essential niyama and yama.

Chapter 2 deals with the essential purification of the nadis. Pranayama is given prominence. Svatmarama presses the relationship between the breath and mind. When the breath is steady, the mind attains steadiness. We are instructed on the technique of *anuloma viloma* pranayama, working with each nostril as the sun and moon, or pingala and ida nadi. This technique specifically includes breath retention, or kumbhaka. The text goes on to teach the stages of purification, including massaging perspiration into the body. We read of the shatkriya, the six acts to purify the physical body in preparation for pranayama, three of which are commonplace and reasonably accessible for the average householder today (neti, trataka, and kapalabhati). The others are certainly approachable for the serious student also. The chapter elaborates on further variations of kumbhaka and multiple pranayama techniques that we still see practiced today. There is brief mention of bandha and pratyahara, with the chapter culminating in an outline of the signs of perfection in Hatha yoga.

Chapter 3 highlights the use of mudras as a means to arouse kundalini. Some of the ten mudras explained are safe for the general practitioner. However, several come with a warning and require the direct guidance from a master teacher. They are all said to assist in halting the decline of the physical body due to aging, along with other benefits. Furthermore, mastery of the mudras is claimed to be a means of attaining certain siddhis. The chapter details some of the intricacies of prana moving into the central sushumna nadi. Finally, the text reminds us of the importance of carefully abiding by the words and directions of the guru.

Chapter 4 aims to illuminate the process of attaining samadhi. Synonyms for this state of being are offered, the common thread being the goal: realizing the Supreme or Brahman. We learn that, through the rise of kundalini and the stillness of mental modifications, karma can be uprooted. Through a sprinkling of metaphor, various methods of moving into the state of absorption are described. This final chapter reveals greater insight into the subtle yogic anatomy, with reference to the granthis alongside the system of nadis. Svatmarama presses that those who choose to remain at the more physical level of Hatha or laya yoga are robbed of the fruits of the path. He gives options for those wishing to attain the ultimate state of Raja yoga. Concentration on nada (sound) through specific techniques—some of which are described in the text—is suggested to be an easy means. In closing, the chapter touches on the state of a liberated being within the world—that is, one who is physically alive but not swallowed up by time, karma, or attachments—that of the jivanmukta.

The Hatha Pradipika outlines a very practical, physical approach toward the path of yoga. It reflects the influence of Tantra through its emphasis on the relationship to subtle anatomy. There are numerous additional classical Hatha texts that are of immense value to any modern-day practitioner. Some noteworthy examples include the *Amaraugha*, *Gheranda Samhita*, *Shiva Samhita*, *Hatha Ratnavali*, and the *Hathatattvakaumudi*.

The study of shastra is meant to be a spiritual practice in its own right. Each text provides its own inner revelations and a deeper esoteric meaning. All too often these sacred yogic texts are read in a "dry" way, without context or meaningful guidance. The teachings only unfold through ongoing study. Quite often it is through a maturation of one's yoga practice that the heart yearns to delve into these sacred texts. Studying the yogic teachings can be experienced as a mystical personal pilgrimage within. Many of the popular yogic scriptures are anchored to some degree in Vedanta philosophy, that is, influenced by the Upanishads. Despite some surface-level conflicts or differences, there is often a common thread binding them all. To embrace the yogic shastra is a very direct way to bring more depth into the practical application of yoga. It is an undeniable invitation to embrace the essence of yoga in everyday life.

There is a sea of rich shastra available for further exploration. Other texts that any sincere seeker may feel called to delve into include the *Ramayana*, the *Ashtavakra Gita*, the *Srimad Bhagavatam*, the *Deví Mahatmya*, the *Vijnana Bhairava Tantra*, the *Amritasiddhi*, the *Saundarya Lahari*, the *Dattatreya Yoga Shastra*, the *Yoga Taravali*, and many more.

CONTEMPLATIONS

Which yoga text featured in chapter five more closely represents the yoga that I have personally experienced or related to?

Which featured text appears to have the greatest value for me to study at this moment on my path?

What are a couple of common threads, if any, that I have noticed through the featured texts?

CONCLUSION

YOGA IS A NOBLE PURSUIT. It is a path of endless sacred study and practice that has the immense potential to uproot or relieve suffering. But not without discomfort along the way. Yoga is not intended to be easy or comfortable all the time. The journey can be confronting and simultaneously offer great boons for those who dare to delve deeply. To be stewards of yoga we must *live* yoga. This is not always an easy task, given that much of yoga today is oversimplified, diluted, and devoid of nuance. It is reasonable to feel lost and lonely when we do not know where to turn or who to trust. Whether you are a practitioner or also a teacher, the pursuit of yoga may feel like a fragile undertaking at times.

Yoga becomes mere exercise or an isolated practice when devoid of the nectar of spiritual principles. In addition, without the cultural context, yoga can feel dry and compartmentalized. To have a foundational grasp on the historical timeline of yoga is the backbone of an appreciation for the intricacies and evolution of the yogic vision over hundreds and even thousands of years. Yoga is a spectrum of techniques and trails to gently tread.

Therefore, while these vast teachings are intended to be transmitted through sound, through speech, and through relationship (the essence of parampara), may this book hold you and offer solace on your journey as a sincere seeker. There is no denying that the yoga tradition at large is one of great knowledge that transforms. This book could never replace the teacher (in all forms) or attempt to traverse the depths of the entire ocean that is yoga. However, I hope that it provides a dependable resource that you will return to repeatedly—with fresh ears and eyes on each occasion. My wish is that it is a wholesome manual that supports your clarity on the context within which all the different techniques and teachings relate to each other.

Take note of the particular aspects of this book that have induced inspiration and enthusiasm. Observe what you intuitively feel pulled to pursue. Perhaps a puzzle piece has now landed in your hands that enables you to experience a sense of renewed certainty or direction, with the faith that the right teacher, text, and teaching will be presented at just the right moment. A commitment to the remembrance and exploration of the subtle anatomy, when engaged in the most physical aspects of yoga, is a rewarding place to begin. Your heart may be summoned elsewhere, however. Importantly, when we yearn for that which is beyond the surface level, we can fall prey to intellectualization as we spread ourselves too wide through the accrual of information. Depth is where the nectar awaits you. Simultaneously, a broad understanding of the systematics, schools, and shastra can promote a frame of reference that helps to uncover the direction we are called to move toward to ultimately approach the depths.

Mastery is gained through consistency, dedication, and surrender. Over time, the practices advance us through a refinement that results in us doing *less*—that is, fewer techniques, less scrutiny, and certainly less dabbling. As we advance along the path, the mind more easily relinquishes control, and we naturally fall into the inward-oriented realms. Over time, as individual dharma is unveiled along with the steady process of resolving accrued karma, we begin to sense where we are headed. The vision and purpose become clearer and are strengthened.

As you honor the desire to uphold the yogic vision, as you crave to drink the nourishment of time-tested wisdom, as you pursue the knowledge that can awaken, may you be divinely guided and held within an aligned community—in *sangha*. My hope is that this book leads you to other sincere sadhakas in the global yoga community who are also steeped in integrity and reverence for the traditions, lineage, and true essence of yoga. Finally, yoga is ultimately a remembrance—or *smarana*. It is a self-remembrance. While a teacher or teaching may assist you in removing the veil, know that everything you need is within you, ready to be revealed. Together, may we always bow deeply in salutations: to yoga, to those who have come before us in yoga, and to the lotus feet of our teachers. It is a tremendous gift to have the fortune to pursue such a virtuous endeavor in this lifetime.

> I am purnam, completeness, a brimful ocean, which nothing disturbs. Nothing limits me. I am limitless. Waves and breakers appear to dance upon my surface but are only forms of me, briefly manifest. They do not disturb or limit me. They are my glory—my fullness manifest in the form of wave and breaker. Wave and breaker may seem to be many and different, but I know them as appearances only; they impose no limitation upon me —their agitation is but my fullness manifest as agitation; they are my glory, which resolves in me. In me, the brimful ocean, all resolves. I, purnam, completeness, alone remain.
>
> OM SHANTIH SHANTIH SHANTIH
>
> —SUMMARY BY SWAMI DAYANANDA SARASWATI[40]

ACKNOWLEDGMENTS

To my dear friend and incredible creative, Tams Hesz—immense thanks for fertilizing the seeds of yoga so many years ago at such a pivotal time in my life. Thank you for instilling a sense of discipline and dedication to the practice and for your friendship, loyalty, and continued care.

Natasha Gilmore, a huge thank-you for your unwavering advocacy—stretching back to my earliest years teaching yoga and now again with this book. Thank you for having my back and for your steady belief. I deeply appreciate your generosity, insight, and professional experience as this book was first coming together. You played a significant part in my vision coming to life. I appreciate having you champion this book early on. Your guidance and responsiveness were greatly reassuring on what often felt like a path of solitude.

To Beth Frankl, executive editor at Shambhala Publications, I felt your sincerity in backing me and this book from day one. Your trust and words of great encouragement have been a remarkable support. I am so grateful you could see the vision and value of this creation and so graciously opened the door to welcome me into this realm of publishing.

Thank you, Samantha Ripley, my assistant editor at Shambhala Publications, for your enthusiasm and attentiveness.

I'm also immensely grateful to Girish Vijayan for thoroughly reading over a significant portion of this book to ensure it was culturally appropriate and respectfully articulated.

To my beautiful children, for your boundless and unconditional love that gives life greater meaning and purpose than ever before, thank you. My love for you is inexhaustible.

And to my husband, thank you for your companionship throughout so many years of evolution—both individually and together.

Notably, I wish to honor and acknowledge the ancient and sacred land from which these teachings have arisen. That is, what is considered in the present day as the Indian subcontinent. Salutations also to the masters and stewards who guarded the nectar of yoga over centuries and beyond so that we can humbly strive toward the highest attainment over lifetimes.

Finally, to the teachers who have profoundly touched my life across various Indic disciplines, my deepest bow to you for your influence and transmission.

Pranamami.

NOTES

1 Paramahansa Yogananda, *Autobiography of a Yogi*, 1st ed. (Philosophical Library, 1946), 214–42.

2 Yogananda, *Autobiography of a Yogi*, 166.

3 Translation by Shantala Sriramaiah.

4 Mahamrtyunjaya Mantra, in Ṛigveda. Personal translation.

5 Nandikeshwar, *The Mirror of Gesture: Being the Abhinaya Darpana of Nandikesvara*, trans. Ananda Commaraswamy and Gopala Kristnayya Duggirala (Harvard University Press, 1917), 13.

6 Charaka Samhita, chap. 1.

7 Robert Svoboda, Living with Reality with Dr. Robert Svoboda, episode 7, "The Four Aims of Life," Be Here Now Network, accessed May 22, 2025, 34 min., 35 sec., https://beherenownetwork.com/living-with-reality-with-dr-robert-svoboda-ep-7-the-four-aims-of-life.

8 Paramahamsa Hariharananda, *Kriya Yoga: The Scientific Process of Soul-Culture and the Essence of All Religions* (Motilal Banarsidass, 2013), 95, 100.

9 Thomas Byrom, trans., *The Heart of Awareness: A Translation of the Ashtavakra Gita* (Shambhala Publications, 1990).

10 Donna Farhi, *Teaching Yoga: Exploring the Teacher–Student Relationship* (Rodmell Press, 2006), 10.

11 Upadeshasahasri (A Thousand Teachings), attributed to Adi Shankaracharya, Prose Part (Gadyabandha), chap. 1 (Shishyaprati-bodhanaprakarana), verse 6. English translation by Kaya Mindlin.

12 Georg Feuerstein, *The Path of Yoga: An Essential Guide to Its Principles and Practices* (Shambhala Publications, 2011), 28.

13 Taittiriya Upanishad, book 1 (Shikshavalli), 11th anuvaka. Personal translation.

14 Donna Farhi, *Yoga Mind, Body, and Spirit: A Return to Wholeness* (Holt, 2000), 7.

15 Pavamana Abhyaroha mantra, from the *Brhadaranyaka Upanishad.*

16 Translated by Baba Hari Dass.

17 James Mallinson, trans., *The Gheranda Samhita: The Original Sanskrit and an English Translation*, (YogaVidya.com, 2004).

18 M. L. Gharote, Parimal Devnath, and Vijay Kant Jha, trans., "Hathatatva-kaumudi: A Treatise on Haṭhayoga" (Lonavla Institute, 2007), 9.13–16.

19 Shandor (Sundernath) Remete, *Taraṇyali Tridhā Dhyānam* (self-pub., Shadow Yoga, 2022), 44.

20 This translation, as well as a handful of others in this book, was based on personal study of Sanskrit and a number of translations.

21 Shandor (Sundernath) Remete, "Nata Yoga," *Shadow Yoga*, accessed September 2, 2025, https://web.archive.org/web/20080618013815/http://www.shadowyoga.com.

22 Baba Hari Dass, trans., *The Yoga Sutras of Patanjali: A Study Guide for Book II Sadhana Pada* (Sri Rama Publishing, 2023), 145.

23 Baba Hari Dass, trans., *The Yoga Sutras of Patanjali: A Study Guide for Book III Vibhuti Pada*, (Sri Rama, 2013).

24 Dass, *The Yoga Sutras of Patanjali.*

25 Yogananda, *Autobiography of a Yogi*, 409.

26 Yogananda, *Autobiography of a Yogi*, 409.

27 Eknath Easwaran, trans., *The Bhagavad Gita* (Nilgiri Press, 2007).

28 John 1:1, Gospel of John, New Testament.

29 Ramana Maharishi, *The Spiritual Teaching of Ramana Maharishi* (Shambhala Publications, 2004), 48.

30 Swami Dayananda, "The Bhagavad Gita," Arsha Vidya, accessed May 22, 2025, https://www.arshavidya.ca/the-bhagavad-gita.

31 Alan Finger, *Tantra of the Yoga Sutras* (Shambhala Publications, 2018).

32 Baba Hari Dass, trans., *The Yoga Sutras of Patanjali: A Study Guide for Book I, Samadhi Pada* (New Age Books, 2010).

33 Finger, *Tantra of the Yoga Sutras*.

34 Edwin F. Bryant, *The Yoga Sutras of Patanjali: A New Edition, Translation, and Commentary* (North Point Pres, 2009).

35 Nischala Joy Devi, *The Secret Power of Yoga: A Woman's Guide to the Heart and Spirit of the Yoga Sutras* (Harmony Books, 2007).

36 Bryant, *The Yoga Sutras of Patanjali*.

37 Baba Hari Dass, trans., *The Yoga Sutras of Patanjali: A Study Guide for Book IV, Kaivalya Pada* (Sri Rama Publishing, 2018).

38 Finger, *Tantra of the Yoga Sutras*.

39 Bryant, *The Yoga Sutras of Patanjali*.

40 Swami Dayananda Saraswati, *Purnamadah Purnamidam* (Arsha Vidya Research and Publication Trust, 2018), 30–31.